Simply Stress

(Stress Management Strategies and Techniques)

Also by Elizabeth J Tucker:
A Simple Guide to Meetings and Minute Taking

Publisher: Shepherd Creative Learning

Simply Stress
(Stress Management Exercises, Strategies and Techniques)

By: Elizabeth J Tucker

Copyright:

First published in 2013
Second edition 2014

Apart from any fair dealing for the purposes of research or private study, or criticism or review, as permitted under the Copyright, Designs and Patents Act 1988, this publication may only be reproduced, stored or transmitted in any form or by any means, with the prior permission in writing of the publisher, or in the case of reprographic reproduction in accordance with the terms and licences issued by the CLA.

© Elizabeth J Tucker 2013
© Elizabeth J Tucker 2014

The right of Elizabeth J Tucker to be identified as the author of this work has been asserted by her in accordance with the Copyright, Designs and Patents Act 1988.

ISBN 978-0-9929479-2-7

Book cover designed by Cassandra Torrecillas -
www.digitallybrewed.com

Copyright © Elizabeth J Tucker 2014

Publisher's Note:

Most, but not all, of the exercises strategies and techniques in this book have been tried by the author. Any views expressed in this book are those of the author.

The author has made every reasonable attempt to achieve complete accuracy of the content in this Guide prior to going to press. The publisher, the editor and the author cannot accept responsibility for any errors or omissions, however caused.

You should use this information as you see fit, and at your own risk. You should adjust your use of this information and recommendations accordingly.

Finally, use your own wisdom as guidance. Nothing in this Guide is intended to replace common sense, legal, medical or other professional advice. This Guide is meant to inform and entertain the reader.

No responsibility for loss or damage occasioned to any person acting, or refraining from action, as a result of the material in this publication can be accepted by the publisher, the author or the editor.

Dedication:

The book is dedicated to Dennis Shepherd (my lovely partner), and Rosemary Tucker and Geoffrey Tucker (my hugely supportive parents).

I've written this book as a result of the death of Dennis in 2012 and my parents in 2008. Both of these situations created unprecedented levels of stress.

Love you all forever.

This book is also dedicated to my amazing friends who have supported me through my stress mountain, and those who prompted the writing of this book. Your friendship is a priceless gift that I shall always treasure. Thank you!

Finally, thank you to Hugh and Sue Price for introducing me to Transcendental Meditation - a worthy investment.

About the Author:

Based near the Cotswolds, Elizabeth has a number of roles. She is a successful business consultant, freelance business trainer, holistic life coach, stress management consultant, mentor, facilitator and author.

Elizabeth is an innovative presenter with an engaging manner. She has a proven track record in helping individuals and organisations achieve their goals. Elizabeth writes her books based on her considerable business knowledge and experience.

She describes herself as an enthusiastic go-getter with a passion for helping others reach their full potential or achieve their goals. Elizabeth uses her own unique blend of insight, wisdom and humour in her work. Her catchphrase is "inspiration and support when you need it".

As well as a successful corporate career she has owned and managed several businesses. Since starting her own business in 2003 she has had the privilege of working with a diverse client base. Her clients have included The Chartered Institute of Housing, blue chip companies, the British Army, charities, social housing providers, SME and start-up businesses, and personal clients.

Elizabeth is currently working on a project to create a series of self-help business books. These will be available as paperbacks and Kindle books. You can find out when these are published by viewing her LinkedIn profile (liz-tucker/10/531/68/) or following her on Twitter (@liztucker03).

Table of Contents

Preface:	10
1. Introduction	**12**
2. Coping Strategies and Techniques	**14**
3. Meditation	**51**
4. Exercises	**66**
4.1 1 Minute Meditation	66
4.2 3 Minute Breathing Exercise (Quick Body Scan)	66
4.3 20 Minutes Hard Work	67
4.4 Anger/Tension Release Exercise	68
4.5 Arms And Hands Deskercises	69
4.6 Autogenic Training Relaxation Exercise	71
4.7 Body Awareness Relaxation Exercise	73
4.8 Cardiovascular Deskercises	76
4.9 Caribbean Beach Guided Meditation	78
4.10 Central Channel Meditation Exercise	80
4.11 Centring Technique Exercise	81
4.12 Chakra Meditation	83
4.13 Chi Visualisation Exercise	84
4.14 Cloud 9 Meditation	85
4.15 Core Deskercises	86
4.16 Deep Breathing Exercise	87
4.17 Empty Mind Meditation	89
4.18 Focused Meditation	89
4.19 Freeze Relaxation Exercise	90
4.20 Giving A Hand Massage	91
4.21 Hand Massage Self-treatment	93
4.22 Heart Centred Meditation	94
4.23 How Stressed Are You? Exercise	95
4.24 Identify Your Coping Strategies Exercise	98
4.25 Legs And Bottom (Gluteal Muscles) Deskercises	100
4.26 Mantra Meditation	103
4.27 Measure Your Current Stress Level Exercise	104
4.28 Mindfulness Relaxation Technique	107
4.29 Mini Self Massage	109
4.30 My Life, My Stress Exercise	109
4.31 Neck Stretch Exercise	112
4.32 Powernap Exercise	113
4.33 Problem Solving Exercise	114
4.34 Problem Solving Visualisation Exercise	115

4.35 Progressive Muscle Relaxation Exercise	117
4.36 Putting Yourself To Sleep Exercise	118
4.37 Put Your Feet Up Exercise	119
4.38 Quick Dealing With Nerves Exercise	120
4.39 Reclaiming Yourself Meditation	120
4.40 Reflective Meditation	121
4.41 Relaxation Exercise For Your Eyes	123
4.42 Relaxation Sequence Exercise	124
4.43 Ritual Departure Exercise	125
4.44 Roll Your Shoulders Exercise	126
4.45 Secret Garden Guided Meditation	127
4.46 Shoulders, Arms And Neck Deskercises	131
4.47 Shoulder Stretch Exercise	132
4.48 Side Stretch Exercise	132
4.49 Stretching Exercise	133
4.50 Taking Control Of Stress Exercise	134
4.51 Taoist Relaxation Technique Exercise	136
4.52 The Calming Effects Of Colour Exercise	137
4.53 The Letting Go Exercise	141
4.54 Visualisation Relaxation Exercise	142
4.55 Walking Meditation	144
4.56 Walking And Writing Meditation	145
4.57 Write A Letter Exercise	146
4.58 Yogic Breathing Exercise	147
5. Conclusion	**148**

Preface:

Pressure and stress seem to be inevitable these days. A little pressure is healthy as it provides the motivation to live a full life. Stress is not good for your physical, emotional or mental health and wellbeing.

Family, friends, colleagues or circumstances may be your stress triggers. However, it is your choice to take stress on board. It may be painful to hear this but, only you can control your stress level. It's no good blaming it on other people.

Nothing can change your life for the better until you take responsibility for your thoughts, emotions and actions. When you do take action you will start to notice some small improvements. The more action you take the greater stress relief you will experience.

Removing stress from your life will take multiple strategies and techniques. It also takes time. Not everyone successfully removes stress from their life. However, we can all reduce our stress level. If you want it enough you will achieve it!

Like everyone else, I've had my share of stress. In fact I've successfully conquered major stress on more than one occasion. I don't claim to have a miracle cure for stress but I believe I can offer you a little help.

I realise that quick fixes aren't long-term solutions. If your stress level is mild a quick fix might be all you need. At other times a quick fix will buy you some time and head space to make longer-term plans. Every small step you take will help.

Much has been written on the subject of stress, and everyone has as opinion about it. So, why have I chosen to write a book on such a popular topic? The simple answer is - when I was at my most stressed I wanted some quick fixes.

Unfortunately, I know a thing or two about extreme stress. In 2008 both of my parents died; just four months apart. Aside from the grief associated with losing my parents I had a lot of other stress at that time.

I turned to my tried and tested stress relief exercises, strategies and techniques. I knew there was no magic wand to make the stress go away. These quick fixes did give me some breathing space though.

I've included each of these exercises, strategies and techniques in this book.

Fast forward to 2012 when Dennis died unexpectedly. This was compounded by a series of events that followed his death. The end result was, at times, an overwhelming level of stress.

Once again I needed to find ways to deal with the day-to-day stress. I worked my way through my existing repertoire. However, on this occasion it wasn't enough. This led me to look for new ways to help me get to grips with the stress I was experiencing.

I was looking for accessible and inexpensive (or free) ways to manage my stress level during this enormously challenging time. I spent many hours looking for additional quick fixes to help me.

I wrote Simply Stress to give you a single point of contact to some short stress relief ideas. When you're feeling stressed you probably don't have the energy or enthusiasm for lots of research.

I would never claim to have a miracle cure for stress. This handy little book contains over 170 stress relief ideas. Each suggestion is intended to provide you with short bursts of respite from pressure or stress.

Most of these exercises, strategies and techniques require no equipment, cost nothing and don't take long to complete. Some you will enjoy and others won't appeal to you. Just choose the exercises that interest you most.

I have deliberately written this book so you can dip in and out of it. There is no need to read it cover-to-cover unless you want to.

Personally, I've found Transcendental Meditation (TM), deep breathing and walking to be the most effective solutions. I do each of these in short bursts each day, and have found the benefits are cumulative.

If you would like to share your success stories with me I would be delighted to hear from you (shepherdcreative0603@gmail.com).

1. Introduction

We would all like to get rid of stress due to the way it makes us feel. Pressure and stress are not the same thing. It's important not to confuse the two.

Pressure is a vital part of life. It motivates us to get out of bed, go to work, pay our bills, do our best etc. Stress is the big, bad wolf we all want to avoid.

The trick is striking a balance where the pressure is acceptable, but hasn't escalated into stress. This is not always easy, but with practice it is achievable. Be kind to yourself, you deserve it.

Each of us has experienced stress at some point in our lives. Most of us convince ourselves that it's an external force beyond our control. Unfortunately, stress is internal and deeply personal to each of us, so we hold the key to resolving the problem.

Family, friends and colleagues may be the cause of some of your stress. Equally, they may offer support when you're stressed, but only you have the power to control it or remove it. This discovery can be either empowering or crushing, depending on your point of view.

The best way to manage stress is to learn some coping strategies that work for you. We all find our own way to do this, so there is no point telling you what to do.

For some it will be drinking, smoking, eating too much (or too little), or taking pills. Some talk incessantly, while others simply withdraw into themselves and bottle things up. All of these are perfectly understandable but they don't make the monster vanish.

There are already plenty of books available that cover the causes and symptoms of stress so I'm not covering these topics. Simply Stress is a compilation of things you might like to try. These are suggestions I found, and tried, to help me cope with my personal stress.

At times my stress felt overwhelming, but I'm glad to say I've survived it. I'm now more resilient to what life throws at me, and have lots of coping mechanisms in my personal arsenal. I've also put measures in place to keep my pressure/stress at an acceptable level.

As a result of finding a permanent solution I can see tangible benefits. I have greater clarity in my thinking; I'm more creative, more productive, and more relaxed. Best of all, I feel so much better for being kind to myself.

Like me, you will find some of these ideas work for you while others don't. That's OK; simply choose the exercises that work for you, or you enjoy doing. To pinch a quote from Tesco - "every little helps". This is certainly the case where stress management is concerned.

If you have never tried any form of meditation before I hope you will have a go. Not everyone takes to meditation straightaway but it's worth sticking with it. Meditation is an excellent tool for long-term physical health and emotional wellbeing. The more you practice meditation the more 'at peace' you will become.

Meditation will help you to view your stressful situations more objectively; rather like a detached observer. This in turn will enable you to be clear-headed and focused when looking for solutions to problems. A clear head is a great way to reduce stress levels.

The exercises, strategies and techniques in this book won't change the situation causing you stress. However, they will enable you to change your reaction and relationship to stressful situations (if you want to).

Although not life changing, these coping mechanisms will provide a temporary stress break. Use this stress break to plan your long-term stress relief strategy. I believe everyone needs their own personal stress management strategy.

If just one message or exercise in this book makes you feel better then it's been worth the investment. The better you feel the more committed you will become to stress management.

"Give your stress wings and let it fly away" - Terri Guillemets (Quotation anthologist)

2. Coping Strategies and Techniques

When it comes to stress management, one size doesn't fit all. Different strategies and techniques work for different people. You may need to try lots of different things before you find the right solution for you.

In this section I have included various coping strategies and techniques. Each has been found to help relieve pressure and mild stress.

None of these coping strategies or techniques are intended to be long-term fixes for dealing with stress. However, each is intended to give you short bursts of stress relief, which can be helpful.

Some of these strategies may work for you, while others might not. Simply choose the ones that interest you most, or try them all and eliminate the ones you don't like.

If you have severe stress related health issues you should consult your GP, or seek other professional medical advice. Never simply ignore your stress symptoms. Unresolved stress can often lead to other physical and mental health problems.

Acceptance:
It sounds too simple to work, but it does. Stop fighting, and learn to accept the things you can't change.

Start by focusing on the things you can change or do something about. Do what you can, and feel satisfied with what you have achieved.

Only then look at the things you can't change. Find your own way of accepting the situation. This will give you a sense of some level of control.

Note: You might like to try the Taking Control of Stress Exercise. By learning the skills of acceptance you will feel less stress and anxious.

Agree With Others (Don't Make Everything A Fight):
Tension and irritability lead to constant arguments. This simply adds to your stress level. Therefore, pick your fights carefully. Ask yourself how much the issue matters to you.

If the issue is not a major one let the other person has their way. In other words - agree with them. There is no point getting stressed needlessly. Not every issue warrants a fight and increased stressed. Save the fighting for the things that really matter to you.

Analyse Your Life:
Do you feel as though your life is in a rut? This can be a comfortable or uncomfortable rut.

Ruts are a major cause of stress. Often we fail to recognise the stress the rut is causing because we are comfortable. You may just feel tired or sad, and not understand why. Chances are you are in a rut.

Take a good long look at all aspects of your life. Be gentle with yourself. As you analyse your life, imagine your conscious mind as a concerned parent talking to a child (your unconscious mind).

Look for creative ways to live your life differently. Alternatively, start a creative project of some kind. Creativity is a great stress reliever.

A Short Brisk Walk And Self-talk:
We all recognise the value of walking. Of course it isn't always possible to take an hour out for a good walk. Don't worry a brisk short walk is beneficial too.

Go for a quick brisk walk. Yes, actually leave the building. I'm sure you've heard the expression "Elvis is leaving the building". Make this your mantra, and just do it.

1. On your way out the door keep saying to yourself, silently or out loud, [your name] is leaving the building

2. Once you get outside say [your name] has left the building

3. Walk briskly for at least 5 minutes. It doesn't matter if you walk somewhere or just walk around the outside of the building

4. As you walk, notice your surroundings, the birds singing or anyone you encounter. Alternatively, recite a mantra. "Life is good, I am great, and I can cope with anything life gives me" is a good mantra

5. After 5 minutes return to work, home or wherever you were before you took this break

Notice how much better you feel after this short break. A brisk walk and self-talk is a great way to clear your head and release anxiety. If you get into the habit of doing this you will find it's a great way to think through problems.

Ask For Support:
For many of us asking for support rates as 'outside my comfort zone'. Although understandable finding someone you can trust to confide in has proven health and wellbeing benefits.

By sharing thoughts you get a fresh perspective. Sometimes we are so locked into our own thinking we can't see the broader picture.

Sometimes a fresh perspective will help. At other times it won't. At least by voicing your thoughts to someone else you don't have to bear the load alone. Make sure you choose someone you trust and whose opinion you value.

1. State your concern/issue. Be factual and specific but don't dramatize. When stressed we have a tendency to exaggerate

2. Tell your listener what you want from them e.g. guidance, an opinion or just a listening ear. If you don't explain what you want they may be tempted to jump into 'fix-it mode'. If this isn't what you want you will just get more anxious

3. Don't expect others to solve your problems for you. This is just a mechanism for you to view the issue more objectively

4. It's important that both of you have the time to commit to this and won't be distracted so ask when it will be convenient to have the discussion

As soon as you recognise that you need help/support ask for it immediately. Don't wait for the wheels to fall off the wagon. Your pressure is likely to increase not decrease by delaying asking for help.

Ask Yourself Empowering Questions:
When we find our back against the wall it's easy to go into victim or blame mode. All this does is increase the pressure; it doesn't solve anything.

Next time you find yourself saying something like "why me?" or "why did I get myself into this mess?" - stop. If you feel like you are having a crisis this is the worst way to fix it.

Instead ask "how can I improve things?" or "what can I do to change the situation?" This subtle change of words will help you to feel more empowered. When you feel empowered you are much more capable of clear thinking.

Beating yourself up will only increase your stress level. Make yourself a promise not to do this again.

Avoid People Who Stress You Out:
We all know people who have a negative impact on us. They may stress your out, drain you emotionally, make you angry, or just leave you feeling down. These are not good people to be around when you are experiencing pressure/stress.

Limit the time you spend with anyone who stresses you out. Being with them will only make you feel worse.

Make a conscious decision not to spend time with them when you are feeling stressed. You might feel guilty initially, but don't give in to these feelings. Put yourself first for a change.

Your stress level will reduce just by not being around negative people. Once you experience this you will find it empowering. This will make the decision much easier next time. I challenge you to try it.

Avoid Unnecessary Conflict:
Are you one of those people who seem to thrive on pitting your wits against others or getting into arguments/disagreements? Stop!

Being needlessly argumentative is not good for your emotional wellbeing. It can be very stressful. If you measure your blood pressure after an argument you will notice it has increased.

A better way to deal with these situations is assertiveness. Look for win/win outcomes where both parties can be satisfied with the outcome.

You still need to use the same creative thinking skills. You are just using them less aggressively, which will help reduce the stress you feel.

Be Inspired:
When you are feeling stressed you probably fail to recognise just how capable you are. When stressed most of us move towards thinking "I can't cope with this". This is really unhelpful thinking.

Instead think about someone who inspires you. This can be your spouse, a family member, friend, colleague or famous person. Create a list of the qualities this person demonstrates and the reason he/she inspires you.

Now look at this list of qualities and identify the ones that you possess. Be honest; don't be too modest.

Next time you are feeling stressed look at your 'Be Inspired' list and be proud of who you are. Tell yourself "I can deal with this" or "I can get through this". If you keep saying positive things to yourself eventually you will believe them. This will pick you up (emotionally) and empower you to find solutions.

Who knows, you may be an inspiration for others sometime. Either way, positive thinking is a powerful stress reduction tool that is often overlooked.

Be In The Present:
You may have heard the expressions "be in the moment" or "be here now". If you don't know what they mean - it's about concentrating on the task you're doing.

Are you one of those people whose mind is always racing? Of course it's great to be able to multi-task, but sometimes you brain would like a short break.

Try this for a change. Whatever task you are doing focus on it completely and don't allow your thoughts to wander to anything else. For example, when washing your hands focus on running the tap, lathering the soap, rinsing and drying your hands.

Don't allow any external thoughts to enter your head for the few minutes this task takes. Initially this may be difficult, but with practice you will soon get the hang of it. Being in the present allows your mind to have a break from being permanently stressed.

Aim to do this several times each day. With practice this will become second nature. As it does, you will feel more relaxed, and so less stressed (if only for a few minutes).

You will find a Mindfulness Relaxation Technique in chapter 4.

Be Near Water:
It is widely recognised that water has a soothing effect on our emotions. It doesn't matter whether it's a water fountain, stream, pond, river, lake or the sea.

Allow yourself to just watch and listen to the water for as long as possible. You will gradually notice your physical and emotional body beginning to relax, particularly if the water is moving.

If all else fails, run a tap slowly for a couple of minutes. Just focus on the water running, and don't allow other thoughts to come into your mind.

Be Realistic:
Perfection is a rare beast, and not achievable when there is a lot to do at one time. We often set unrealistic expectations of ourselves and others. This just adds to the pressure we're feeling.

It's common to think I/he/she could have done better, but this is counter-productive. Be realistic, it's better to do a good job on time than a perfect one late. While you are busy striving for perfection other tasks will fall by the wayside.

If you can learn to develop realistic expectations you will feel less stressed. Lots of good results are better than one perfect outcome.

Brain Download:
Do nagging thoughts or problems distract you from the task at hand? If so, this is probably putting a little extra pressure on you. Try this instead. Carry a notebook or keep a list on your smartphone.

Every time something gets in the way of what you are trying to do, make a note of it. This acknowledges the thought but allows you to forget it until you can give it your full attention.

Break The Destructive Cycle:
Negative thinking is both destructive and contagious. Eventually negative thoughts become a self-fulfilling prophecy. This increases rather than decreases stress.

It may take a few weeks but you can break this destructive cycle. Try the following:

1. Each time you have negative thoughts about one of your stressors/stressful situations put 50 pence or £1 in a money box

2. Psychologically this will raise awareness each time you give stress the upper hand. You will be conscious of having to forfeit money for every negative thought. It's a bit like having a swear box for negative thoughts

3. You can break this habit quickly by being conscious of what you're doing. It's widely accepted that a habit can be formed in 21 days. Equally, habits can be broken

4. You will know you have conquered the destructive cycle when you stop paying forfeits

5. When you stop putting a forfeit into your money box use the funds to treat yourself to something nice

Centring:
Centring is a technique that originated, and is still used, in Aikido. At its most basic level, stress is a form of energy like any other. Centring is a process that helps to manage energy; including stress.

This exercise takes 20-60 minutes. It involves deep breathing, concentration and imagination. You will find instructions for centring under the Centring Technique Exercise in chapter 4.

Challenge Yourself And Grow Your Confidence:
There is a link between self-confidence and stress. The less self-confidence you have the more vulnerable you feel. Vulnerability often contributes to stress.

I'm not suggesting that being self-confident will automatically make you stress free. This would be far too simplistic. However, greater self-confidence does help loosen the grip stress has on you.

Setting yourself goals and challenges helps to build self-confidence. This can be work related or personal. For example, you could try learning a new language.

Your new found confidence will equip you deal with stress better. Professor Cary Cooper is an occupational health expert at the University of Lancaster. According to him "by continuing to learn, you become more emotionally resilient as a person. It arms you with knowledge and makes you want to do things".

Complete One Thing At A Time:
Do you seem to be permanently juggling to keep lots of balls in the air? If so, you are actually adding to your pressure/stress level.

You will feel better if you do one thing at a time. Finish one task, no matter how small, before moving onto the next one.

By allowing yourself to finish something you will have a sense of achievement. This sense of achievement will give you a feeling of control. A sense of control is helpful for reducing stress.

This is such a simple idea, but a very effective one.

Control Email Stress:

The evolution of technology seems to be driving us to be constantly connected to our emails and other devices. This makes us less, not more, productive.

It's important to give your brain a rest if you want to maintain peak performance at work. Therefore, don't allow work/business emails and calls to impinge on your time outside work.

Switch off your laptop, ipad, mobile phone (and any other devices) when you are at home. Your employer pays for your working time, not family or leisure time. Enjoy quality time not focusing on work-related matters.

Your brain needs this down time. Your reward will be greater clarity and efficiency, enabling you to maintain peak performance at work. Try it for a couple of weeks and notice the difference.

Control Your Environment:
You may not have full control over your environment; particularly at work. For instance, you can't choose the office colour scheme or layout.

There are still small things you can do to create the right environment for you. Here are some suggestions you might like to try:

1. Place your favourite photo or picture on your desk
2. Declutter your desk space
3. A desk tidy (for your pens etc) in your favourite colour. Never choose a colour that you don't like
4. Notepads with pretty pictures or patterns
5. Coloured pens
6. Repositioning your PC or telephone etc
7. A plant or some flowers

Little things make a difference. If your environment feels good your stress level will be lower as you will feel generally calmer.

Counselling:
Many larger employers offer a professional counselling service to their staff through an employee assistance scheme. This confidential, professional service is paid for by the employer. Find out if your employer offers this scheme.

It can help you find ways to cope with stress and deal with the causes of your stress. It doesn't matter whether your issues are personal or work related. Your employer is never given the details of your discussions.

This is a valuable perk that many employees don't use. Having someone independent and non-judgemental to talk to can be hugely beneficial to your emotional wellbeing.

Create A Personal Attributes List:
If you were asked to describe the attributes of one of your friends you could probably do it easily. Describing your personal attributes is often much harder.

Being a friend to yourself is important to your emotional wellbeing. The more you like yourself the more comfortable and relaxed you will be in your own skin.

We often find it hard to list our personal attributes, and yet we find it easy to say why we like our friends. This exercise is about being a friend to you.

Make a list of all your personal attributes. Your list should be a minimum of three entries, but ideally 10 or more. Whenever you feel stressed, or in a negative mind-set, simply look at your list. Better still, try adding to it.

The concentration this exercise requires removes you from your negative mindset temporarily. This will improve your state of mind, and so your ability to cope with stress.

Crying:
For a very long time we heard expressions like "don't cry" or "stop crying". Now scientists and medical practitioners are moving away from this stance.

More and more we are now being told about the healing power or tears. Obviously we do shed tears at extremely happy events. However, most tears are shed as a result of stress, sadness, grief, anxiety or frustrations.

When you're stressed your body creates adrenaline and cortisol. The more stressed you become the more of these chemicals your body creates. The build-up of these chemicals then makes you feel worse.

Tears are the body's release valve. Crying releases some of these chemicals that have been stored in your body and brain.

The act of crying is natural and cathartic. It's a great way to purge pent-up emotions. This act of cleansing your mental and emotional state restores balance and harmony.

You may not feel on top of the world after crying but you will feel somewhat better. I'm not suggesting you resort to crying about everything, but don't try to stop yourself having a good cry. Sometimes it's exactly what's needed.

Crystal Healing:
When people talk about crystal healing do you immediately imagine new age mumbo jumbo? Crystal healing has been around for centuries. Like everything else it has varying degrees of success, but it's certainly worth a try.

Crystals are particularly good at helping us adapt to changes in energy frequencies created through stressful situations. Small crystals can be worn as jewellery or placed in pockets etc. Larger crystals can be placed on your desk or somewhere else.

It is believed that having a large crystal in a room can help reduce stress, by reducing negative energies and harmonising imbalanced energy patterns.

Personally, I keep a smoky quartz on my desk to protect myself against stress and frustration from co-workers or clients. I also keep a rose quartz and amethyst close by. When I'm feeling tense I hold one of them in my hand for a few minutes.

You will find lots of information on the internet regarding Crystal Healing.

Cycling:
Cycling is great for blowing away the cobwebs. It can help you to make decisions and push through mental blocks. The flow of oxygen to your little grey cells fires up the neurons. This provides some space from the pressures of daily life.

"Saddling up and hitting the road releases natural feel-good endorphins. This helps counter stress and makes you happy" according to Jenny Edwards CBE (CEO of the Mental Health Foundation).

Dealing With Nerves:

It's a fact, we all get nervous, but what can we do about it? We have a tendency to believe that nerves always work to our detriment. This is not true.

Nerves give you an adrenalin rush and give you the desire to perform well. I believe this is a good thing. On the converse side, unnecessary nerves lead to pressure and stress. This is counter-productive as you then fail to perform at your optimum level.

When you're feeling nervous your automatic reaction is often fight or flight. Sometimes, but not always, this is useful. I believe it's important to get the balance right.

A constant attack on your nerves leads to anxiety. When anxiety takes its toll your body knows it. You may have trouble sleeping, eating and/or concentrating. At worst, you may have panic attacks.

I'm sorry to say there is no silver bullet, but you can learn to work with your nerves. The basic antidote is to work on your internal compass. The idea is you should stop caring so much about what others think and focus more on what you think.

There is a relatively new thinking that suggests we should learn to read and respond to situations:

Step 1: Try to read the situation as objectively as possible. The key to this is not to rush to respond

Step 2: Go through a cognitive process of understanding the consequences of your response. By taking the time to think about the consequences it may encourage you to respond differently.

Obviously this is not a quick fix. This is a behaviour that needs to be learnt over a period of time. In the short term try the Quick Dealing With Nerves Exercise.

Declutter:
We don't always recognise clutter as a stressor, but it certainly can be. Never underestimate the effect that clutter can have on you.

Mess/clutter creates confusion and a sense of powerlessness. At its most extreme, clutter can be completely overwhelming. If you have seen the TV programmes about the hoarders you will realise the detrimental effect clutter has on people's lives.

If your home, car or desk is messy and disorganised declutter it. This will instantly make you feel as though you are more in control. A sense of control (no matter how small) can help reduce stress levels.

Deep Breathing:
There is now considerable clinical research that suggests there are tangible benefits to deep breathing.

This is something you can do anywhere anytime, and it only takes a few minutes (so there's no excuse). Just five minutes deep breathing will set you on the path to better physical and mental health. So, what are you waiting for?

See the Deep Breathing Exercise for instructions. If you need a little help there are lots of deep breathing apps you can download. Some are free and others you need to pay for. I'm sure there is one that will suit you.

Delegate:
We tend to assume that delegation is something our manager does at work. Sometimes it doesn't occur to us that we can all adopt delegation skills.

Learn to use delegation skills at work and at home. You can delegate upwards as well as downwards. Delegating even the smallest task can have a positive mental effect. To get you started:

1. Create a list of all the things that need to be done (at home or at work)

2. Identify which tasks **you** need to do yourself

3. Now identify the tasks that someone else could do for you (be honest with yourself). You really don't need to do everything yourself

4. Finally, identify the tasks that don't really need to be done at all, and then ditch them

5. Assertively (not aggressively or passively) allocate tasks to colleagues or family members. Be positive not hesitant. This suggests you're expecting them to comply and so you'll encounter less resistance

Deskercise:
Deskercise is a catchy name given to exercises that you can do at your desk. Deskercises are short bursts of exercise for the desk bound or those, like me, who hate the gym.

You will find deskercises under Arms and Hands, Cardiovascular, Core, Legs and Bottom (Gluteal Muscles), and Shoulders, Arms and Neck Deskercises. Why not try a few or all of them.

If you are feeling stressed a few minutes deskercise will increase your metabolism. This will help to put you into a more positive mindset, which is essential if you want to conquer stress.

Distraction:
It's generally accepted that distraction can be a simple but effective de-stressor technique. It works because your mind is focusing on something other than your stressors.

Find an activity that you can absorb yourself in. Do this for 5-20 minutes. Afterwards notice the changes in your mindset.

Try to build distraction into your life several times a week. Over time you may choose to do longer distraction activities.

Don't Start The Day In A Mad Rush:
Do you start every day in a mad rush? Do you feel you have to hit the ground running from the moment you put a foot out of bed? Stop! You're putting yourself under pressure before your day even starts. This means the rest of your day will follow suit.

Even if you have to get up slightly earlier, allow yourself the luxury of a slightly slower start. This will make you feel more in control. Even the smallest amount of control over your life is a stress management technique worth mastering.

Do Something Creative:
Doing something creative is a great way to reduce stress.

Whether you are naturally creative or not you may find an activity that you like. This could be knitting, writing poetry, creative writing, gardening, painting/drawing, or anything else you fancy. Perhaps you can find something that you can involve your family and friends in - a win/win outcome.

If your work doesn't involve creativity it's even more important to build a little creativity into your week. Have fun experimenting. Who knows what new talents you may discover.

Eat Nutritious Food:
I don't want to preach, but eating nutritious food has its part to play in stress management. This doesn't have to be expensive. Make an

effort to add one healthy addition to your diet each week. Alternatively, cut out one unhealthy item each week.

A healthy diet will make you feel better. When you feel good stress seems much more manageable.

Exercise:
Although exercise can be beneficial it doesn't mean you have to go to the gym or take up jogging to get physical activity into your life.

Being active helps improve how your body works and improves your state of mind. Think about the physical activity you already do as part of your day-to-day life:

Vacuuming

Going up and down the stairs (at home or at work). Try to increase the number of times you do this each day

Doing the grocery shopping or having a retail therapy day. You will be surprised at how far you walk

Lifting and moving your children (if you have a young family) or adults (if you care for an adult family member)

Going for a walk

Gardening

Horse riding

Cycling

Skipping

Simply try to add a little more activity into your life. This can be something as simple as getting off the bus one stop earlier, or walking to the shop for your sandwich at lunchtime.

Feel The Fear And Do It Anyway:
Yes, I've used Susan Jeffers famous quote "feel the fear and do it anyway".

The first step to addressing your fears is to acknowledge them. Also acknowledge the stress your fears cause you. This is a positive step forward. The next step is to create an action plan. Make sure your action plan consists of small manageable steps.

When your action plan is complete look at what you have achieved. Feel a tremendous sense of achievement and satisfaction.

Whenever you achieve something, big or small, feel empowered. This in turn leads to stress reduction.

Get Some Fresh Air:
Just a few minutes fresh air is good as it's a great mood lifter. Even if you don't have time to go for a walk you can benefit from a few minutes fresh air.

1. If you're stuck in the office all day, try standing on the doorstep every couple of hours and take 4-5 deep breaths. Just fill your lungs with fresh air and notice how you feel

2. With each deep breath smell the atmosphere. This could be the trees, rain, flowers, traffic fumes, or anything else. It really doesn't matter; just stimulate your sense of smell

3. When you feel ready go back to what you were doing

This short wellbeing boost may be all you need to get you back on track.

Note: You can do this at home or at work.

Give Yourself A Hug:
Hugging is an extremely positive form of communication. It also has health benefits. Hugging lowers blood pressure, which is one of the main risk factors of heart disease.

Hugging relieves stress. It releases Oxytocin, the hormone that makes you feel calmer and less anxious. Hugging also releases serotonin and dopamine. These hormones make you feel good and lift your mood.

It might seem strange to give yourself a hug but give it a try and see how you feel.

Research by Dr Kristin Neff suggests it's as beneficial as a hug from someone else. She says your brain responds to the hug not the hugger. When you feel low or stressed, wrap your arms around yourself for a quick hug.

Give Yourself A Treat:
Don't save the celebrations for large victories. Reward every small victory with a treat. Treats don't have to be big or expensive. Recognising each achievement, even with a small reward, will lift your mood.

Your reward could be 10 minutes reading a book/magazine, a chocolate or something more expensive and indulgent. The choice is yours. Rewards create a positive mind-set. This in turn helps to reduce stress.

It's important not to feel guilty about the treat. Treats only have a positive effect on your mental state as long as you don't immediately feel guilty about what you've done.

Gratitude:
A lot has been written on the power of gratitude. It's one of the greatest ways to develop feel good emotions.

In case you're reading this and thinking 'my life is awful, what have I got to be grateful for?' Stop! Everyone has something to be thankful for. You're alive; that's something to be grateful for.

Set yourself a target of spending at least five minutes every day contemplating all the things you have in your life. This is called developing an attitude of gratitude. It will help you to view situations more positively.

Positive thinking is widely accepted as a useful contributor to stress reduction.

Hand Massage:
Physical contact is a basic human need. Just like hugging, your brain will happily accept a hand massage from you.

This can be a couple of minutes or much longer, but the act of massaging your hand/arm is very soothing. This has the psychological benefit of providing self-nurturing. The calmer you feel the more able you are to deal with stressful situations.

See the Hand Massage Self-treatment for instructions. You will find this in chapter 4.

Have A Cup Of Tea:
Have a cup of tea - this might not seem like a stress reduction strategy. We now have proof from Scientists at UCL that a cup of tea reduces cortisol levels. Cortisol is a stress hormone. If you needed an excuse for a tea break, you've got one now.

Hum A Tune:
Sing or hum your favourite feel-good song. Don't worry that you don't have the voice of an angel. Most people don't.

Singing helps lower the level of Cortisol (stress hormone) in your body. Singing shifts your mental activity from your left brain to your right brain.

Anything that lifts your mood is helpful to stress management.

Humour:
Humour is one of the greatest and quickest devices for reducing stress. Best of all, it costs nothing.

Humour works because laughter produces helpful chemicals in the brain. According to Loma Linda University in California, stress hormones are reduced by 70% when we laugh.

Humour gets your brain thinking and working in a different way. It distracts you from having a stressed mind-set. Distraction is a simple effective de-stressor technique that takes your thoughts away from the stress, and thereby diffuses stressful emotions.

Most people will feel different and notice a change in mind-set after laughing and being distracted by something humorous. Why not practice your best 'dirty old man laugh'! Remember, laughter is infectious.

Identify Your Fabulous 15:
You may have 500 friends on Facebook or 500+ contacts on LinkedIn, but these are not the people who make a real difference to your life.

Identify the 15 people you cherish most. These are the magic people who bring joy, wellbeing and satisfaction into your life. Make space for the magic 15 in your life. These are the people you can turn to in moments of pressure, stress or trauma.

Improve Your Communication Skills:
Assertiveness is a skill that everyone can benefit from. Learning assertiveness skills will give you useful techniques for all aspects of your life.

Assertiveness is far less stressful than being aggressive or passive. It will also help you to maintain a general sense of wellbeing.

You might like to have a go at a short assertiveness quiz to find out how assertive you are. If so, have a look at www.stress.about.com. In the search box, type 'The Assertiveness Quiz'.

Join A Self-help Group:

You may be able to find a self-help group. You can talk to someone in the same boat as you, or at least understands what you are going through.

If your issues are more general you may find it helpful to call the Samaritans. Their service is free, confidential and available 24/7. Sometimes talking to a stranger while you remain anonymous can be very helpful.

It really doesn't matter who forms part of your support network. The important bit is making sure you have access to the help and support you need.

Keep In Touch With Friends:
You may not always have time to go out with friends but it is important to keep in touch. This keeps the connection and provides you with a reliable source when you need someone to talk to. Ways to stay in touch:

1. Each week ring, email or text your friends. This shows you are thinking about them, and don't just get in touch when you have problems

2. At least quarterly, make time in your diary for a face-to-face contact. This can be a quick drink, going to the cinema, meeting for dinner or anything else you fancy doing

3. Be there for your friends. They need support too

When a crisis hits get in touch straightaway. The sooner you get help/support the less stressed you will feel.

Know Yourself:
We all think we know ourselves, but how much do you really know? Most of us spend so much time just getting on with things we fail to analyse our strengths and weaknesses.

1. Think about the things you do well or enjoy doing (at work and at home)

2. Identify your weaknesses, or the things that cause you stress

3. Identify the tasks that you can delegate to others (at home and at work)

4. You now know where you need help. Arrange training to plug your skills gap or find another strategy to deal with the tasks that cause you stress. For example, delegate the tasks you aren't good at

The more confident you feel the less stressed you will be. Remember, only you think you have to be good at everything.

Lark Or Night Owl:
Do you know whether you are a lark or a night owl? Most people are at their most productive in the morning (lark) or late afternoon/evening (night owl). It can be helpful to know your peak performance time.

First, identify if you are naturally a lark or a night owl. Next, try to do the tasks that take most effort during your peak performance time. You will find this less stressful.

Don't try to constantly force yourself to do complex tasks at your lowest performance time. This simply increases your stress level and further reduces your productivity.

By managing you time around your body clock you will be more productive and less stressed. A win/win outcome.

Lend A Listening Ear:
We can all benefit from having someone who will lend a listening ear. It's important to be a giver as well as a receiver.

You don't need to be a professional counsellor in order to be a good listener. If you want to be a good listener and support your family, friends or colleagues apply the following rules:

1. Let the other person speak without interruption

2. Give them time – don't rush them. Sometimes people are slow to start talking, but once they get going the floodgates seem to open

3. Ask open questions to move the discussion on

4. Don't give an opinion unless you're asked to. Remember – sometimes people just want a listening ear

5. Help the other person distinguish the facts from the emotions. This can be tremendously helpful in stressful situations

6. Provide a different perspective. Sometimes this is all that is needed

You might like to follow-up at an appropriate time to see how they're getting on.

Never underestimate the value of a listening ear. It has a part to play in a long-term stress management strategy.

Make Friends With Aromatherapy Oils:
Since prehistoric times aromatherapy oils have been used to promote physical, mental and spiritual wellbeing. The most common psychological benefits of aromatherapy are spirit stimulation, mental clarity, stress relief and mood improvement.

Pure essential oils are generally massaged into the skin, but they can be inhaled or used in baths. Massage enables the essential oil to be absorbed into the bloodstream. This produces physical therapeutic benefits.

When an essential oil is inhaled it activates the nerve cells in the nasal cavity. This sends impulses that stimulate the brain and produce positive feelings and emotions.

If you can afford it, book an aromatherapy massage and be prepared to feel very relaxed afterwards. Otherwise, buy a bottle of aromatherapy oil and inhale it to help keep your stress level manageable.

Make Time For Fun And Relaxation:
Never underestimate the value of time for a little fun and relaxation. When you are feeling stressed you probably feel as though you can't relax. Also, fun probably feels like the last thing on your mind.

This is exactly when you are in greatest need of a little fun and relaxation. Your mind and body need a little nurturing to maintain balance.

Think of the things you enjoy doing, and try to build at least one into your schedule each week. The more fun you have in your life the less stress you will experience.

Manage Your Time:
Poor time management skills often contribute to stress levels. There are lots of good training courses available to help you master good time management skills.

We all believe there are too few hours in the day. Instead of focusing on the lack of time available, focus on what you can achieve in the time you have. If you can't afford a time management training course try this instead:

1. Write a list of all the tasks you have to do today, this week or this month. This can be work or home related tasks

2. Identify your priority tasks. Don't fall into the trap of convincing yourself that everything is a priority

3. Now identify the tasks that could be delegated to someone else

4. You should now be left with a list of less important tasks. Identify the ones that don't really need to be done, and ditch them

Psychologically several small lists are less stressful than a single long list. Instead of getting stressed because you aren't super human, accept the world won't end just because some things don't get done. Accepting you can't do everything is both liberating and stress relieving.

Mantras:
At the mention of the word mantra some people immediately think new-age or religion and switch off. Please don't dismiss mantras without first considering their merit.

Repeating a mantra stimulates the pineal and pituitary glands (among others), and so creates health benefits.

A mantra is a single word or short phrase that is repeated for several minutes, or even hours. Mantras are often used in meditation, but you don't need to meditate to successfully use mantras.

Generally mantras have no meaning. It is simply a word or phrase that creates a vibration through repetition. It's like plucking the string on a guitar or violin and allowing the vibration it creates to spread through your body.

A mantra is often used to break into our thoughts and create a calmer and more relaxed state of mind.

For more information, please refer to the Mantra Meditation.

Media Fast (Unplug) For A Day:
A growing trend in the US is spending a technology free day. This means no TV, radio, smart phone, ipad or laptop.

You may find the idea of a media fast scary. Research shows that those who try it genuinely feel better at the end of their media fast.

Why not set aside one day each month as a media fast day. After all many generations before us existed quite happily without being plugged in.

Meditation:

Meditation is a deeply relaxing mental and physical activity. It allows you to separate yourself from your thoughts and feelings temporarily.

The purpose of meditation is to slow your mind down and allow you to find some stillness and peace. Think of meditation as a stress-reduction break.

Meditation has proven physical and mental health benefits. These include:

1. It decreases your respiratory rate
2. It increases blood flow and slows your heart rate
3. Regular meditation leads to a deeper level of relaxation
4. It helps reduce blood pressure
5. It can help reduce anxiety attacks
6. It decreases muscle tension and headaches
7. It increases serotonin, which influences your mood and behaviour. Lower levels of serotonin are often associated with depression, obesity, insomnia and headaches

There are various forms of meditation. If you haven't already experienced meditation why not give it a try. I have included a chapter on meditation as it's gaining in popularity.

Mindfulness:
Mindfulness is an age-old technique, but it has recently become a hot topic, and the latest fad. I hope this enthusiasm doesn't fade as it requires little effort and costs nothing.

There are lots of definitions of mindfulness. These include - the gentle effort of being continuously present with the experience. Or, paying attention is a particular way, being in the present moment. There are many more definitions but hopefully you've got the idea.

There is ever more research linking mindfulness to stress reduction. Research suggests that mindfulness decreases the level of the stress hormone cortisol. It often forms part of yoga practices, but mindfulness can be a stand-alone activity.

For more information, please refer to the Mindfulness Relaxation Technique.

Never Dwell On Mistakes:

What is your attitude to mistakes? Do you learn from them and move on, or do your beat yourself up? The latter simply adds unnecessary stress.

It's a fact; we all make mistakes. Learn something from every mistake as this will turn a negative experience into a positive one. If you repeatedly think about, and overanalyse, past mistakes stop! This action is stressful, and a waste of time.

Nurturing:
Nurturing is a basic human need. It's not frivolous; it's a necessity to maintain a sense of physical and mental wellbeing.

If you make nurturing a part of your schedule you will have a better mindset to deal with life's stressors. Here are just a few nurturing suggestions that you might like to consider:

1. Read a book, magazine, newspaper or e-book reader
2. Take a short nap or meditation
3. Spend time outside enjoying nature. This could be watching the birds in your garden, sitting quietly, fishing, going for a walk, or anything else you enjoy doing
4. Call a friend for a chat
5. Light scented candles and inhale the aroma
6. Take time to savour a cup of tea or coffee
7. Work in your garden for a short period
8. Listen to your favourite feel good music
9. Watch a comedy
10. Take a weekend or short break away

Don't get so caught up in the hustle and bustle of life that you forget to take care of your own needs. Self nurturing is a necessity, not a luxury.

Pamper Yourself:
Believe it or not; pampering yourself is good for your physical and mental wellbeing. Do you have so many responsibilities that you forget to take care of yourself? Self-care is an important aspect of stress management.

Each person's idea of pampering is different. Pampering suggestions include having a massage, a reflexology treatment or any other holistic therapy, having a manicure/pedicure. It could even be soaking in a warm bath for five minutes longer than normal.

Identify what pampering means to you and build it into your daily life. Pampering is about taking time out to care for you. It will revitalize you inside and out. A more positive mental state enables you to be more productive and take care of those who depend on you.

I hope you are now convinced that pampering is a necessity, not a luxury you don't have time for.

Pet An Animal:
Studies have identified that petting an animal can improve a person's psychological and physical health. Petting an animal is known help in the reduction of blood pressure.

We all know the benefits of having a good friend we can share our problems with. Recent research suggests that spending time with a pet may be even better. One of the key benefits is the animal doesn't talk back, it just listens.

Just by petting an animal you can relieve tension and calm your nerves. You don't have to own an animal to do this, but Psychologists are encouraging us to make contact with animals.

Research suggests that even watching a goldfish can have a calming effect on some people.

Physical Activity:
Work off your stress. Any kind of physical activity has emotional wellbeing benefits.

You don't have to go to the gym or go jogging to benefit from physical activity. A walk, cycle ride or a swim will also release negative energy just as effectively.

Try to build a little more physical activity into your life. Afterwards, notice how much more relaxed you feel. This will motivate you to incorporate more physical activity into your life.

Powernap/Catnap:
Do you often find yourself hitting a slump in the middle of the afternoon? If so, a powernap or catnap may be just what you need. Margaret Thatcher was famed for the powernap.

A quick nap is nature's way of recharging and re-energising your body. A powernap/catnap of 10-30 minutes is believed to help reduce stress temporarily. Don't feel guilty. We all need different amounts of rest to operate at our best. Learn to listen to your body.

If you would like to try a powernap you will find details under the Powernap Exercise in chapter 4.

Practice Saying 'No':
Do think of 'NO' as a dirty word? All too often we want to say no but find ourselves saying yes instead. It's important to remember that you have needs too so don't feel compelled to say yes to every request.

Saying yes when you should be saying no often creates unnecessary stress. It's important to understand why you always feel compelled to say yes. The common reasons for finding it hard to say no are:

1. You want to help
2. You're afraid of appearing rude
3. You're a people pleaser
4. Fear of conflict
5. Fear of lost opportunities. Perhaps you are worried about closing doors on future opportunities
6. Some people view 'no' as a sign of rejection

If it feels better, say 'no' and then follow it up with your reason for saying 'no'. It's important to be assertive not aggressive or passive when saying no. Remember, it's not personal. You are saying no to the request, not the person.

Prioritise/Plan:
Learning to prioritise and plan tasks can be beneficial in stress reduction.

Never underestimate the value of a 'to-do' list. A 'to-do' list is a simple time management technique that anyone can adopt. It will help you to get organised and efficient at completing tasks.

A 'to-do' list is a way to quickly and effortlessly get into the habit of time management like a professional. Best of all, it takes very little time and costs nothing.

Try the following for a month and then see how much more efficient you are. Also notice the contribution it has made in reducing your stress level:

1. Before leaving work each day write tomorrow's 'to-do' list. This allows you to forget about tomorrow's tasks when you leave work. It is essential to give your brain some down time if you want to maintain optimum performance

2. At the start of the day review your 'to-do' list and split it into what you must do today and what can be done another day. This simple task will take a little pressure off you

3. Cross tasks off as you complete them. Psychologically this will give you a sense of achieving something

4. Don't be tempted to write a new 'to-do' list each time you complete a task. This is simply wasting time and puts you under additional pressure

Problem Solving:
For some bizarre reason when we are feeling stressed we try to solve all our problems at once. This simply makes us feel even more stressed.

Developing your problem solving skills can help you to develop strategies to manage your stressors. It's a powerful tool to add to your stress management toolbox.

Don't simply write an endless list of all your problems as this may overwhelm you. Instead think of a single problem that you would like to tackle.

Identify the problem, focus on the issues (but don't look to apportion blame), and then look at what you can do about it.

For more information on problem solving, please refer to the Problem Solving Exercise in chapter 4.

Punctuate Your Day With Pauses:
Do you lunge straight from one activity to another? Instead of taking a five-minute break do you find yourself planning what you will do next? If so, stop! This is adding to your stress level.

At the end of each activity allow yourself a five-minute break. You could do five minutes of deep breathing, stop for a 'mindful' cup of tea or coffee, stand on the doorstep and get some fresh air. The list is endless.

The point is - make this a ritual. At the end of each activity take a five-minute break before starting your next task.

This is a very quick and easy habit to adopt, but it will send a switch-off signal to your brain. Even this small pause in your day will provide wellbeing benefits.

Put Things Into Perspective:
It sound very simplistic, but when we are feeling stressed we generally lose our sense of perspective. This simply makes matters worse and increases the stress level.

Show yourself a little kindness and put things into perspective. Next time you are feeling overwhelmed and losing your sense of perspective try the following:

1. Write the facts of the stressful situation down on paper. This is just the facts, not the emotions you're feeling about the situation. This will clarify your thinking and help you to see the situation in different ways

2. Put yourself into someone else's shoes. This can be a family member, friend or colleague. How might he/she perceive the situation?

3. Talk to other people. Share your concerns and ask for their perspective of the situation. You may not agree with their opinion, but it will help you to see the situation from a different perspective

4. Now review your perspective of the situation. Do you feel less or more pressure? Generally people feel less pressure once they have looked at the situation from various perspectives.

This won't always work but it's worth a try as it costs nothing and only takes a few minutes

Quality Time With Your Loved Ones:
Sometimes the thought of spending time with your family and loved ones can be stressful. However, recent research suggests that being surrounded by those closest to you can relieve stress.

Perhaps you work long hours. Maybe you feel tired when you get home and have little time or energy for your loved ones. These are the most important relationships in your life so don't neglect them.

You may not have a lot of time together so make sure the time you do spend together is 'quality time'. It will give you a sense of wellbeing, which is a natural stress reducer.

Read A Book, Magazine, Newspaper Or e-Book Reader:

How often do you read for pleasure? We have so much required reading in our everyday lives that sometimes we forget how enjoyable reading for pleasure can be.

Reading can be a wonderful (and healthy) escape from everyday life. A study at the University of Sussex found that reading can reduce stress by 68%. It's also believed to work better and faster than listening to relaxing music or drinking a hot cup of tea.

According to Dr David Lewis, reading for just six minutes can reduce stress. What are you waiting for, here's the perfect opportunity to have a six minute stress break.

Rehydrate:
Most of us fail to drink enough water. We seem to be far happier drinking tea, coffee, fizzy drinks, 'sports' drinks, fruit juice or alcohol.

All of your organs, including your brain, are strongly dependent on water to function properly. The human brain is 90% water, so it stands to reason that it needs regular rehydration to maintain peak performance.

Drinking enough water can help improve your mood, which in turn often helps reduce stress. If you starve your body of water your ability to function well will be reduced. Try drinking 4-8 glasses of water daily to remain hydrated.

Sleep:
The amount of sleep needed varies from person to person. Sleep is often recognised as a de-stressor as it's a chance to relax.

We all know that people in the Mediterranean and Central Americas take a siesta every day. This is almost certainly linked to longer life expectancy and lower levels of heart disease.

Have a notepad beside your bed. If you think of something in the middle of the night, write it down. This will allow your brain to go back to sleep, rather than having to remember your thought. Having to remember your night time thoughts interferes with your sleep.

Too much sleep can make you feel as bad as too little sleep so let your body tell you what it needs.

Slow Down:
Are you one of those people who always seem to be in a rush? If so, you are probably making your mind and body feel tenser as you're not allowing yourself chance to relax.

When we're tense we often find ourselves doing things faster than normal. All you need to do is allow an extra minute.

Be aware of what you're doing (be in the present) instead of doing everything on automatic pilot. Here are some typical examples of where you can slow down:

1. Having a shower
2. Washing your hair
3. Getting dressed
4. Rushing to get into the car
5. Driving to work
6. Having breakfast
7. Watering the garden
8. Walking the dog

Slow down, observe what you're doing and then be still for 10 seconds before you resume your normal activities. Practice this every day for a week and notice how much better you feel.

Stop Procrastinating:
Have you noticed that when you feel stressed or anxious you procrastinate? Unfortunately, this simply adds to your stress level, it doesn't remove the problem.

Tackle challenges as soon as you become aware of them. Set yourself small achievable goals. As you achieve your goals you will develop a feeling of achievement and satisfaction. This is a great motivator and so a good way to address procrastination.

The only time procrastination is beneficial is if you use the delay to objectively assess the situation and plan your solution.

Stress Diary/Journal:
For many, a stress diary or journal is an effective stress management tool. Like every stress management tool or strategy, this won't be the right solution for everyone.

Keeping a daily stress diary or journal works for those who don't want to share their problems with others. If you are going to use a stress diary/journal you need to do so for at least 28 days.

Aim to write in your stress diary/journal for at least 10-15 minutes each day. Write down what is causing you stress and how you feel about it.

At the end of your 28 day period review what you have written. Look for any daily stress patterns, explore your stress thoughts and look at your stress coping skills. Finally, identify any negative behaviour patterns.

Use your findings to create a longer-term stress management strategy or plan.

Take A Break:
Don't use the excuse "I haven't got time for a break". In truth, you can't afford to not take a break if you want to take care of your physical and emotional wellbeing.

A short break of 10-15 minutes is all that is needed. This is long enough to give your brain a rest, and will significantly improve your performance. You will come back refreshed and will easily make up the time used to take a short break.

Take A 'Mindful' Shower:
Mindfulness is a hot topic currently. Suddenly everyone seems to be commenting on the benefits of mindfulness in all aspects of our lives.

Researchers at the University of Pennsylvania found that focusing on the tasks we usually hurry through can reduce negative emotions. One example was taking a shower.

Next time you take a shower focus on the sensations, smell and sounds around you. Feel the water rushing over you instead of planning the rest of your day.

In other words, enjoy the here and now instead of constantly looking ahead. This won't take any longer than normal, but it does allow you to enjoy your shower for a change.

Take Stock:
Taking stock is just about taking a very short break for a quick self-assessment.

Build a little 'taking stock' time into your daily schedule. Ideally, you should aim to take 2 minutes in the morning and 2 minutes in the afternoon. Even this short burst of taking stock time can be beneficial to your emotional wellbeing.

During the break ask yourself "how am I doing?" and "are there any areas of tension in my body?" If so, address them immediately.

Building these short breaks into your daily schedule will help you to manage your stress level better, and make you aware of any potential health issues.

Talk Therapy:
Humans have been communicating through speech for 80,000 years. Talking about the things that are bothering you helps create clarity and get things into perspective.

You may choose to talk to family, friends, healthcare professional, counsellors, the clergy, the Samaritans, or anyone else. There are three types of talk therapy. These are cognitive, behavioural and interpersonal.

Cognitive talk therapy helps you change harmful ways of thinking. Behavioural talk therapy helps you change harmful ways of acting, and interpersonal talk therapy helps you relate better with others.

Initially you may find it hard to talk openly about personal issues. Therefore, talking is a skill that needs to be learnt like any other. This act of discussing your feelings will enable you to gain a new insight and perspective. It can be very beneficial to stress management if you allow others to help you.

You will find information about Talk Therapy on the internet. Simply type 'Talk Therapy' into your search engine.

Taoist Relaxation Technique:
The Taoist Relaxation Technique is a breathing technique. This technique is known to have many health benefits. It improves circulation, increases performance, reduces stress and can help you cope with negative emotions.

Experts claim that if you do this exercise daily you will start to notice changes within a week. I have included the Taoist Relaxation Technique Exercise in chapter 4 if you wish to try it.

The Calming Effects Of Colour:
Colour therapy, chromotherapy, is not as commonly known or understood as other forms of therapy. Simply put, different colours can positively (or negatively) alter your emotions, mood and overall wellbeing.

Colour contains an electromagnetic energy. Every colour seen in the rainbow contains its own healing property. Therefore, it stands to reason that colour has a part to play in stress or stress relief.

The earliest recording of colour therapy dates back 2500 years; just in case you believe it's some new age phenomena.

On a non-conscious level we respond to colour. The easiest way to incorporate colour into your life is consciously choose the colours you wear each day. For example, did you know that dark blue has a calming effect on the body?

If you're interested in studying colour therapy there is lots of information available on the internet. I have included The Calming Effects of Colour Exercise in chapter 4.

The Quiet Garden Movement
The quiet garden movement campaigns for the provision of peaceful public places for personal reflection. Spending time alone in a beautiful setting may be all you need to restore your sense of balance and wellbeing.

Solitude is often undervalued. However, it's a free, simple and effective antidote to stress. Imagine it as your personal inner monastery - a place where you can retreat to when you need to find peace.

Why not create your own solitude space at home. Simply put a chair in a quiet corner of your home and tell everyone this is your 'quiet place'. Retreat to this space when you need a little peace and solitude.

Time/Spontaneous Natural Improvement:
Time is the most neglected of all stress treatments. When we're stressed we automatically assume we must find a solution. In reality mild stress sometimes rights itself if you give yourself time and be kind to yourself.

Time, as a stress reducer, is likely to work if you're in the first stage of stress. It can also work if you're receiving practical help and/or emotional support from family and friends. Six to 12 weeks is the norm for this spontaneous natural improvement.

Time/spontaneous natural improvement doesn't work for everyone. If you don't see or feel any improvement after 12 weeks you may need to seek professional help or find a different solution.

Use Positive Affirmations:
Affirmations are statements that give you conscious control of your thoughts. We already know that thoughts create our reality. So, it makes sense to use positive rather than negative affirmations as a stress reduction tool.

An example of a negative affirmation is "I'm broke; I never earn enough to have a decent lifestyle". A positive affirmation might be "I'm really good at my job, I do it well and I enjoy working here".

Become aware of the messages you're sending to yourself. The sooner you do this the sooner you will achieve a happier and calmer state of mind.

If you find yourself constantly making negative affirmations it follows that your beliefs about life will be negative. This will increase your stress level. Start practising positive affirmations to train your subconscious mind towards a more positive state.

On post-it notes write down any inspiring messages or expressions that you come across and can relate to. Stick these messages somewhere you can see them e.g. fridge, PC, office wall etc. Read them regularly until you naturally develop a positive mindset.

You may like to write yourself a personal daily positive affirmation. I post a positive affirmation on Twitter every day. If you'd like to sign up for these messages you can follow me on Twitter @liztucker03.

Use Scent To Improve Your Mood:
Some scents generate a feeling of calm, while others may remind you of romance. Equally, some may signal danger to you. Either way, scent is a powerful natural mood enhancer. The right scent at the right time can be helpful in reducing stress.

Certain aromas are believed to activate the brain's feel good chemical, Serotonin. All you need to do is drip a few drops of your chosen scent onto a tissue.

Jasmine, lavender, clary sage, chamomile, neroli and vetiver aroma therapy oil are all good for stress management. Simply sniff the tissue whenever you feel stressed.

Visualisation For Problem Solving:
Whether we're aware of it or not we often use visualisation to solve problems. Sometimes we create an image of the situation that is

bothering us in order to make sense of it. Sometimes we find ourselves overanalysing the problem, which isn't helpful.

Athletes often use visualisation to help them succeed in their chosen sport. The benefits of visualisation as a stress management tool are widely recognised. It only takes a few minutes and can quickly make your feel more relaxed.

I have included a Problem Solving Visualisation Exercise in chapter 4 if you want to have a go at it. There is also plenty of information available on the internet if you want to know more.

Volunteering:
Volunteering might not be your first thought when you're feeling stressed. However, volunteering can be an excellent stress management strategy. Volunteering works because it takes you away from the situation causing you stress.

Anything that emotionally removes you from your stressor is good. You will come back to the problem with a fresh pair of eyes.

There are lots of different volunteering opportunities available. Decide what you're interested in doing and then approach the organisation.

Walk For Headspace
A walk puts mental and physical space between you and a stressful situation. It also gives you time to think and reflect. Research shows it can induce calm by prompting the release of chemicals that stimulate relaxation.

You can walk alone or with others, it costs nothing and you can do it anywhere. What are you waiting for? Even a short walk will make you feel better.

What Can I/Can't I Control:
An effective way to control stress is to identify what you can and can't control about the situation. The key to success is learning to accept the things you can't control. Each of us will find our own coping mechanisms, but it's helpful to know what yours are.

If you or a family member is facing redundancy, you can't control that. However, there are things you can do.

If redundancy is likely, get your CV up-to-date. Also practice interview techniques and questions, identify your core skills and which skills you would like to use. Finally, identify potential sources for finding work if you are made redundant.

Even a small amount of control does help in stressful situations.

Work Less, Succeed More:
I'm sure you've heard of 'working smarter not harder and SMART targets'. When these expressions first started being bandied about it was assumed this was just another fad. Not so.

Now business gurus agree that working harder doesn't automatically get better results. They suggest that working constantly with no change of pace, task or scene is the enemy of creativity and innovation.

If the rational, decision making, part of your brain works too hard for too long it simply becomes depleted.

Vary your tasks. Don't stick at the same task too long. Also remember to take regular short breaks. A comfort break or taking a break to make a tea/coffee gives your brain chance to regroup. This will enable you to go back to the task fresher.

Cut yourself some slack and work smarter not harder. If you push yourself too hard you will cause yourself unnecessary stress and reduce your productivity.

Worst Case Scenario:
Inside all of us is a hidden Drama Queen. Your internal Drama Queen may not appear very often, but she is lurking there in your subconscious.

If you are not a natural Drama Queen you may find this only surfaces when you are feeling stressed. Have you noticed - when you're feeling stressed everything seems much worse?

The best way to tackle this is to give your mind free reign for a short time. Just allow yourself to imagine the worst case scenario.

1. Imagine the worst-case scenario. Imagine the situation being worse than it really is. Write down all your 'worst case scenario' thoughts. You will feel better after you've done this

2. Now consider the very best outcome (also known as blue sky thinking) you can imagine. Write down what this would be. I know this sounds fanciful but do it anyway

3. Next, consider what the most likely (realistic) outcome is, and focus on that

4. Now take a reality check. In the great scheme of life (the bigger picture) how important is this issue?

In three months' time is it still going to be as important to you? Does it warrant the pressure you're putting yourself under? Do you have a tendency to put yourself under pressure for things that aren't really that important?

5. Talk to yourself firmly, but kindly, and reassure yourself that you can deal with the situation. More importantly, know with certainty you can deal with this

Once you have completed this exercise you will be able to return to your normal self.

Write A Letter:
Metaphysicians have proved that thoughts can create emotional clutter. When you're feeling stressed your brain seems to become completely absorbed in the person or situation causing you stress. It then feels impossible to battle your way out of the situation.

Sit down and write a letter. If it's another person causing your stress, write a long, detailed letter to him/her. Say everything in this letter you probably would never say to their face. Get rid of all your pent up emotions on paper.

If it's a situation that's causing you stress, write a letter to yourself. Tell yourself all about the situation and how it makes you feel. Make your letter as detailed as possible.

When you have finished your letter burn it. Now let your thoughts and emotions go. This exercise is believed to be a good way to release stress and emotional intensity.

Yoga, Tai Chi, And Qi Gong:
Each of these ancient Chinese healthcare systems combines exercise, breathing and meditation. Yoga, Tai Chi, and Qi Gong are all recognised as a useful technique for physical and mental wellbeing.

There are many different types of yoga, tai chi and qi gong so you have plenty to choose from. Do a little research to find which one suits you best, and to find your nearest class. This information is readily available on the internet.

Your Coping Strategies:
You may have your own coping strategies, which aren't included in this book. Why not write them down as a reminder for yourself next time you're feeling stressed.

If you would like to share your coping strategies I would love to hear from you. Please email me at shepherdcreative0603@gmail.com. Alternatively, you will find me on LinkedIn (liz-tucker/10/531/68/).

Zumba:
Zumba is a dance fitness program created by dancer and choreographer Alberto "Beto" Perez in Colombia during the 1990s.

Zumba involves Latin and international music with dance moves. The routines incorporate interval training (fast and slow rhythms) and resistance training.

If you're feeling energetic, Zumba can be a great stress buster. If you're more couch potato than fitness fanatic Zumba probably isn't for you.

Personally, I haven't had a go at Zumba as being a 'sweaty Betty' holds little appeal for me. It seems to be like marmite - you either love it or hate it!

"It's not stress that kills us; it's our reaction to it" - Hans Selye (an early pioneer of the modern stress theory. His scientific research helped to shape our understanding of stress)

3. Meditation

As meditation is such a large topic I've given it a chapter on its own. There is sufficient information available that I could write a book on the subject. Instead I have chosen to give you a flavour of some of the most popular types of meditation. I hope this will whet your appetite.

There are hundreds of different meditation techniques. Meditation is practiced by people from all walks of life. The group I meditate with consists of a solicitor, psychiatrist, and other business professionals, a housewife, retirees and students. Meditation is available to everyone.

Nowadays more and more medical professionals are recommending meditation to their patients. They recommend meditation for a variety of medical conditions as well as mental and emotional wellbeing.

Meditation is believed to help - insomnia, anxiety, stress, blood pressure and help asthma patients to breathe more easily.

Personally, I find regular meditation gives me greater clarity in my thinking and encourages creativity. Both are very useful when it comes to writing.

Meditation is a safe and simple way to balance your physical, emotional and mental wellbeing. Whichever type of meditation you opt for the fundamental principles are the same. These are:

1. During meditation your mind should be focused on now, not the past or future

2. If you want to gain benefits from meditation it should be practiced regularly, not as a one-off exercise

3. Meditation creates clear awareness, not the type of normal awareness that human beings experience. This can be beneficial to every aspect of your life

4. The human mind is thought to have five important faculties. These are - confidence, effort, mindfulness, concentration and wisdom. Meditation helps to balance each of these

The true benefits from meditation come from quality not quantity. Devotees of meditation report they are able to find greater peace, happiness and freedom from suffering. All of these significantly contribute to stress reduction.

Meditation is also used in yoga practice, although you don't have to practice yoga to meditate. Meditation can successfully be used as a stand-alone activity. Personally, I've been practicing various forms of meditation for over 15 years. However, I've never done any form of yoga.

Meditation is almost indispensable in today's fast paced world of strife and competition. Regular meditation will reward you with lower levels of pressure and stress.

I'm not suggesting that you need to spend several hours a day meditating. Even if you just do a few minutes each day, over time you will notice some tangible benefits.

It has been scientifically proven that meditation is good for us physically, mentally and emotionally. You may choose to do your own research on the many benefits of meditation. The list is endless!

If you just want a quick summary to help you decide if meditation is for you here are my findings:

1. Meditation induces deep relaxation, which is key to successful stress management

2. Meditation increases the oxygen flow to your brain. This is turn enables clearer thinking, better reasoning skills, greater awareness and perception

3. Meditation improves blood flow to your muscles. This will give you greater stamina

4. Meditation slows your breathing down. This contributes to a decrease in asthma attacks

5. Meditation deepens your spiritual awareness. This in turn generates greater understanding, tolerance and patience

6. Meditation relaxes the autonomic nervous system and lowers your heart rate

7. Regular meditation practice leads to greater self-awareness

8. Meditation helps practitioners to remain calmer in the face of drama

9. Regular meditation increases the production and release of serotonin (a feel good chemical)

10. Meditation can help prevent or reduce panic attacks

11. Meditation improves memory skills. It can also be helpful when you are trying to learn something new

12. Some advocates believe meditation increases intelligence

13. Regular meditators often report they have greater problem solving skills, particularly complex problem solving

14. Meditation helps promote assertive behaviour, rather than aggressive or passive behaviour patterns

15. Some report that meditation helps in the fight against addiction (drugs, alcohol and smoking)

16. In general, regular meditators find it easier to fall asleep and benefit from better quality sleep

17. There is some evidence that meditation helps reduce cholesterol levels. This is linked to lower blood pressure levels

18. Meditation is available to everyone. Most meditation costs nothing, requires no special equipment and can be done anywhere

19. Meditation strengthens will power and inner strength

20. Meditation shifts brain activity to less stress prone areas of your brain. This decreases the negative effects of mild stress, depression and anxiety. Some people find it helps them to avoid depression

21. Regular meditators report a decrease in physical pain

22. Meditation reduces inner turmoil and mind chatter

23. Meditation is known to increase energy levels and mental endurance

24. Over a period of time, meditation is known to lower levels of heart disease

25. Meditation enables your body to return to a status of calm after a fight or flight reflex. It also brings about calmness after a row, argument or physical attack

26. Meditation increases your immune system. This helps ward off physical ailments and diseases

27. Meditation can be used in conjunction with conventional medicine and holistic therapies

28. Meditation helps promote mindfulness. It reduces your desire to live in the past, or fretting about the future

29. Meditation helps promote positive thinking. This is useful for overcoming obstacles and achieving your goals more easily

30. Meditation improves your digestive system

31. Meditation neutralises any tendency to mood swings

32. It has been found that hand-eye coordination improves with regular meditation practice

33. Meditation positively affects the aging process (physical and mental)

34. Meditation brings about permanent positive benefits with regular practice

35. Just 20 minutes twice daily is sufficient to benefit from meditation

To ensure fairness and balance I have researched the negative side-effects of meditation. Although there are some negative side-effects there are far less of these than there are benefits. I have captured the most common ones for your information.

The first thing to say is meditation can be a frustrating process in the early days. Not everyone takes to meditation like a duck to water. For some the learning process can be slow and hugely frustrating.

New meditators often report feeling agitation initially. Some meditators find it difficult to sit without moving, for up to 20 minutes.

Some meditators report wanting to keep checking the clock to see if they have finished their 20 minutes meditation. If you experience this, why not start with five minutes and build up to 20 minutes.

Not everyone is comfortable sitting in a lotus position. Don't worry, you don't have to. Sit on the floor (with a cushion underneath you). Alternatively, sit on a comfortable chair to do your meditation. Sitting comfortably is essential if you want to reduce the chances of agitation.

Meditation is 'me-time'. Some meditators say they feel guilty spending time on themselves. They also report family members feel resentful that meditation time means less family time.

You could make meditation a family event, where you all meditate together. Put things into perspective, you are only giving yourself 20 minutes me-time twice a day. This really isn't a great indulgence.

Fear is an emotion that some new meditators experience. Meditation brings you in touch with your deepest self, which can raise some issues you didn't want to face. The best way to deal with this is to acknowledge your fears, but don't engage with them. Just act like a casual observer watching a film. Don't form an opinion on what you are seeing.

It's important for your physical, mental and emotional health to deal with your inner demons. Over time meditation can be a very effective way to deal with old issues. It's important to be kind and gentle with yourself as this can be a painful process.

You may need to try various different options until you find the right one to help you address your inner demons.

The only other significant issue I've come across is finding the right type of meditation for you. There is not a 'one size fits all' style of meditation.

You may need to try several different types of meditation before finding the one that suits you best. Rather than getting frustrated with the process, enjoy experimenting.

Whichever type of meditation you choose grounding is important. It's a good idea to get into the habit of grounding yourself after every meditation. Choose one of the following ways to ground yourself after your meditation practice:

1. Slowly drink a glass of water
2. Have something to eat. Don't eat a heavy meal as you will find it hard to digest right now
3. Have a shower
4. Stamp your feet
5. Have a quick catnap

"Being a detached observer as the scenes of life pass by will enable you to understand the secrets hidden within" - Brahma Kumaris.

Below you will find a summary of the most popular types of meditation. I hope this will help you to identify which types are best for you.

Body Scan Meditation:
Body scan meditation is great for anyone who is looking for a quick form of meditation. It can be a short burst (3-5 minutes) or a longer meditation if you prefer. See the 3 Minute Breathing Exercise (Quick Body Scan) and Body Awareness Relaxation Exercise.

Body scan meditation is also good if your mind tends to wander during meditation. During this meditation you focus on the sensations and feelings in different parts of your body. This distracts you from other thoughts.

Breath Watching:
This is also known as Deep Breathing Meditation. As the name suggests, this type of meditation is about being aware of your breath while meditating. See the Deep Breathing Exercise.

This is a very easy form of meditation to master. You can do it anywhere and at any time e.g. sitting at your desk, on the train etc. This meditation can be done with your eyes open or closed; the choice is yours.

Central Channel Meditation:
If you are a meditation beginner this type of meditation might suit you. This is an ancient Taoist method, which has been modified for modern times.

Instead of focusing on your breathing you focus on a beam of energy entering your crown. This is known as the 'medicine palace'.

You feel the beam of energy flowing in through your crown as you begin to inhale. You then follow your breath down through your energy channels (chakras) to the sacral chakra.

Finally, you follow the energy back up the central channel and out through your crown as you exhale.

After practicing this type of meditation some people report their head or whole body shakes. Don't panic. This is a sign of the effectiveness of your meditation practice.

Chakra Meditation:
Chakras as the energy centres positioned vertically throughout your body. Each of the seven chakras is responsible for controlling the flow and distribution of energy in your body. The seven chakras are (from the base) - root, sacral, solar plexus, heart, throat, third eye and crown.

An imbalance in one or more of your chakras may result in physical, mental or emotional wellbeing issues. Chakra meditation focuses on restoring the balance of these energy centres.

Chakra meditation works with each chakra in turn, starting with the root chakra. Each chakra governs a particular element of your life. This type of meditation systematically works through all the elements of your life.

Your chakras are located in the following areas of your body:

1. Root chakra (red in colour) - this is situated at the base of your spine. It is located at the tail bone in the back and the pubic bone in the front. The root chakra is good for grounding you and keeping you connected to the physical world. It also works on stability and the male fertility

2. Sacral chakra (orange in colour) - this is situated two inches below your navel. It is routed in your spine. This chakra focuses on creativity and female fertility

3. Solar Plexus (yellow in colour) - this is situated two inches below your breastbone. It is in the centre of your body, behind your stomach. This chakra works on self-will, confidence and self-worth

4. Heart chakra (green or pink in colour) - this is situated behind the breastbone. It is on your spine between your shoulder blades in the back and behind the breast bone in the front. This chakra works on romance, self-love and affection for others

5. Throat chakra (blue in colour) - this is situated in the 'V' of your collar bone in your lower neck. This chakra focuses on all elements of communication

6. Third eye chakra (indigo in colour) - this is situated above your physical eyes in the centre of your forehead. This chakra focuses on intuition, perception, psychic ability and a balanced state of mind

7. Crown chakra (violet in colour) this is situated just behind the top of your skull. This chakra focuses on spirituality and giving you peace and wisdom

I have included a chakra meditation in the next chapter.

Empty Mind Meditation:
As the name suggests this type of meditation requires your to empty all thoughts from your mind. The idea is to allow your mind to empty and just rest. This allows peacefulness to take over.

Personally, I find this type of meditation quite challenging. It's actually quite difficult to empty your mind of all thoughts, and not allow thoughts to drift into your mind. If you are new to meditation, this is not the easiest meditation to start with.

Focused Meditation:
This is sometimes referred to as Simple Meditation. This type of meditation focuses on something. This can be music, an object, a

mantra or a single thought. Most commonly people focus on an ornament or candle flame for this type of meditation.

Relaxation music is helpful for this type of meditation. Even if you're focusing on an object or thought having music playing quietly in the background is soothing. If thoughts pop into your head simply refocus on your chosen object etc.

You will be amazed at how rejuvenated you feel afterwards.

Guided Meditation:
A guided meditation involves being led through a relaxing imaginary environment. Ideally you want someone with a soothing voice to guide you through this style of meditation.

As the speaker describes a place or journey in great detail you visualise it. By concentrating on the speaker and the visualisation your mind is having a break from your issues or thoughts. If the speaker has a soothing voice you will find this is a very relaxing form or meditation. Also, you won't notice time passing.

I have included two guided meditations for you to try. See the Caribbean Beach Guided Meditation and the Secret Garden Guided Meditation. There are also lots of free and paid-for apps that you can download.

Heart Centred Meditation:
This is sometimes referred to as the Heart Chakra Meditation. Throughout this meditation you focus on your breathing and use a ball of healing love energy to heal yourself. See the Heart Centred Meditation for instructions.

Your body pumps 4.4 million pints (2.5 million litres) of blood each year. Aside from working hard, it also reacts adversely to pressure and stress. Your heart deserves a little kindness.

The purpose of this type of meditation is to release your fears and any sadness you feel. These emotions are then replaced with loving kindness and compassion.

Heart Rhythm Meditation (HRM):
This type of meditation focuses on your breath and heartbeat. You focus on your heart as the centre of your energetic system. At the same time you make your breath full, deep, rich, rhythmic and balanced. HRM creates a state of balance between your head, heart and emotions.

Fans of this meditation state that if you practice this regularly you become compassionate, more sensitive and more powerful.

This meditation takes approximately 10 minutes to complete. The heart rhythm meditation is an audio-led meditation. You will find it by logging into http://www.healthy-heart-meditation.com.

Curtis also runs a 7 week heart meditation rhythm e-course. You will find details by using the same link.

Journey Meditation:
Journey meditation involves visualisation. If you are someone who finds visualisation easy you will probably enjoy this type of meditation.

You start off by writing down all the things that cause you anxiety, tension or fatigue. You can then choose which ones to deal with during your meditation. You can choose how to deal with the others later.

Next you have two choices. Option one is to close your eyes and focus on one or all of these stressors. Keep meditating and having peaceful thoughts about the stressor(s) until you feel de-stressed.

The other option is to close your eyes and just focus on feeling peaceful. Once your meditation is complete you will feel much better able to cope.

Kundalini Meditation:
Kundalini meditation isn't a belief or religion; it's simply a technique to help you gain inner peace.

Kundalini is an energy that exists in everyone's body; usually in a dormant state. Kundalini meditation awakens this sleeping state and enables practitioners to reach high levels of spiritual awareness.

This can be an incredibly powerful type of meditation but it isn't everyone's cup of tea. If you would like to know more about this type of meditation type 'Kundalini Meditation' into your search engine. You will find lots of information readily available.

Many people notice side-effects after Kundalini meditation. Side-effects include - a tingling sensation in your head, a change in body temperature, muscle twitching, pinched nerves/muscles or an energy burst. Some also report spontaneous uncontrolled movements and back pain.

Mantra Meditation:
This is also referred to as vibration meditation. Mantra meditation is a chant meditation. Either loudly or silently you chant a single word or short phrase repeatedly.

'Om' is a popular word used in chant meditation. Repeating the word 'Om' over and over creates a deep vibration. As you meditate you focus on this vibration, which then induces deep relaxation.

The more you practice this style of meditation the more aware you will be of sinking into a deep state of relaxation. You will find instructions for this type of meditation under Mantra Meditation.

Mindfulness Meditation:
This has greatly increased in popularity recently. Mindfulness isn't new; it's an age old Buddhist tradition. Mindfulness just seems to be one of the buzz words for 2014.

Buddhists call mindfulness Vipassana or insight meditation. Mindfulness is the ability to experience what you're doing currently without your mind filling with other thoughts.

This technique may feel difficult to grasp initially, but with practice everyone can master it. You might like to try the Mindfulness Relaxation Technique in the next chapter.

As you meditate you will continue to hear the noises around you. You will also feel the sensations and have a general awareness of everything that is happening. Imagine yourself as a casual observer. You see, hear and feel but you don't form any judgment about any of it.

Mindfulness has long-term physical and mental wellbeing benefits. Meditations involving mindfulness have long been used to reduce stress. Some require focusing your attention on a single thought. Others encourage your to follow and then release your thoughts and feelings.

Movement Meditation:
Most people prefer to do movement meditation when they are alone, unless they practice it as part of a meditation group. It requires you to lose yourself in movement. Fans of movement meditation say it can be extremely uplifting and relaxing at the same time.

You sit comfortably with your eyes closed and focus on your breathing. Once your breathing is stable and rhythmic you begin the movement. A slow swaying motion is easy to do if you want to try this type of meditation.

Alternatively, you might prefer to dance. Simply find some slow, soothing, music and try some gentle dance moves. Lose yourself in your fluid dance moves and forget the world around you. Do this for as long as you want to.

Qi Gong:
This is another Taoist form or meditation. Qi Gong uses your breath to circulate energy through your organs and energy centres (chakras).

During this type of meditation you focus attention on three major energy centres. These are your sacral chakra, heart chakra and third eye chakra.

Your sacral chakra is located two inches below your navel. Your heart chakra is in centre of your chest, and your third eye chakra is in the centre of your forehead.

If you log into Google Play (https://play.google.com) you can download a Qi Gong Exercise and Meditation App. This is a free App showing different Qi Gong exercises and meditations. They are designed to help you achieve perfect inner balance, strength and calm.

Reflective Meditation:
This is sometimes referred to as an Analytical Meditation or the Mastermind Meditation. It's all about disciplined thinking.

In order to successfully practice reflective meditation you need to choose a word e.g. joy. Then you explore your word in great detail.

The key is to just focus on thoughts associated with your chosen word, and not allow other thoughts into your mind. This is a good mind training exercise but some find it boring.

Initially your mind may wander to other thoughts and topics. If this happens you just bring your mind back to your chosen word. If you practice this type of meditation every day your mind will become more in control. Over time your mind will stop wandering off.

Reflective meditation is considered to be one the most important types of meditations. Many believe it has a long-term calming effect on the mind.

Reflective meditation stimulates transformative power. It provides great conviction and strength to change the course of your life. This is a good type of meditation for self-disciplined people. If you would like to have a go at this, see the Reflective Meditation in the next chapter.

Simple Meditation:
This is sometimes referred to as Focused Meditation. As the name suggests this is simple to do. It's a good starting point for anyone who isn't accustomed to sitting and focusing on a particular object for long periods.

Simply find a peaceful place to sit and find an object you can focus on. Spend 10-20 minutes focusing on this object. A candle flame is a popular choice as it's easy to watch the flame flickering.

Initially thoughts may pop into your head. Don't try to hold onto these thoughts, or engage with them. Acknowledge your thoughts and allow them to come and go.

Spiritual Meditation:
This is sometimes known as Prayer Meditation. It is often practised by those who regularly participate in prayer. It's based on communicating with your God (or the creator).

Say your prayer and then tell God/the Creator what your problem is. Often the answer will be presented to you in prayer. This is why people often refer to their prayers being answered by God.

Transcendental Meditation:
This is generally referred to as 'TM' by meditators. TM claims to be the purest, simplest and most effective form of meditation the world has known. The great thing about TM is anyone can do it, with very little effort.

This is gaining in popularity and is widely being recognised by medical professionals. There is considerable research into the health benefits of TM.

Its popularity is also partly due to celebrities like Russell Brand and David Lynch endorsing it. If you would like to know more, simply type 'Transcendental Meditation' into your search engine.

TM requires repeated chanting of a sacred word. You are given this sacred word as part of your induction ritual. TM needs to be learnt by attending a training event from a certified TM teacher.

There is an initial cost implication, but personally, I believe this is an investment worth making. If you are considering learning TM, simply attend a free introductory talk. At the end of it you will be asked to decide if this is the right meditation for you. You will not be put under any pressure.

Details of your nearest TM centre can be found on the TM website (http://uk.tm.org). Note: TM is practiced and taught throughout the world so wherever you live you will be able to access a TM teacher.

The Mail Online featured an interesting article on 4 June 2014 that you might be interested in reading. Here is the link to this article - http://www.dailymail.co.uk/sciencetech/article-2648556.

Vibration Meditation:
Also see Mantra Meditation for this type of meditation. Vibration meditation is a mantra meditation, which involves repeating a particular word or sound. As you do this you create a vibration, which passes through your body.

This vibration induces a state of relaxation. This is why meditation is such a key element in stress reduction and stress management.

Visualisation:
This is sometimes referred to as Creative Meditation. It's somewhat different to other types of meditation. The aim is to consciously strengthen different qualities of your mind.

This type of meditation focuses on strengthening appreciation, joy, compassion, patience, empathy, love, gratitude, humility, fearlessness and tenderness. It's also used to help people develop self-belief.

Some of the world's most successful people, including great athletes, swear by visualisation. It's also often used to achieve personal success and for creating abundance.

Simply put, visualisation uses the power of mental imagery to achieve your desired outcome.

In order to achieve great success with this type of meditation you first have to still your mind. Once you can move beyond worries, anxiety, stress, depression or fatigue you end up with crystal clear thinking and mind mastery.

This type of meditation may sound difficult to master, but it isn't. Start with a few minutes each day and simply build up your meditation. Once mastered, you can get into a creative meditation state easily. I have included a Visualisation Relaxation Exercise in the next chapter.

Walking Meditation:
This type of meditation involves consciously focusing your mind on walking. It can be difficult to master initially, but with regular practice it can be very beneficial.

It involves focusing on your feet and legs. Each time your mind drifts away from your feet you have to refocus on the act of walking. As you walk notice the sensations you feel in your feet and legs.

It's a good meditation to do as it gets you outside. It's an opportunity to get some fresh air and appreciate nature. I have included two Walking Meditations in the next chapter.

Yoni Mudra:
This is a slightly different style of meditation. This involves using your fingers as you breathe.

During this meditation you close your ears with your thumbs. Then you use your index fingers to cover your eyes and your middle fingers to pinch your nostrils. You press your lips together with your remaining fingers. While meditating you release your middle finger as you inhale and exhale.

Personally, I'm not a great fan of this type of meditation. To me, it feels unnatural and uncomfortable. I will leave you to make up your own mind about Yoni Mudra.

Zazen Or Zen Meditation:

This is a generic term for seated meditation in the Buddhist tradition. It is often referred to as 'just sitting'.

This is not a quick meditation; it is done over long periods of time. It requires you to sit on a zafu or small pillow. You sit with your back straight, ideally in the lotus position, for several hours at a time.

This type of meditation was developed for a monastic setting. It doesn't fit naturally with an active life. If you have the time and ability to do this type of meditation it is said to uncover hidden awareness within you.

As I stated at the start of this chapter, there are hundreds of types of meditation. Hopefully, I have given you enough options to encourage you to give meditation a try.

I've been practicing different types of meditation for many years. I generally do this twice a day, for 20 minutes. Sometimes I do a much longer meditation if I feel my mind and body need it. I simply allow my mind and body to tell me what it needs.

"Meditation is painful in the beginning but it bestows immortal bliss and supreme joy in the end" - Swami Sivananda (one of the greatest yoga masters of the 20th century).

4. Exercises

In this chapter I have included a selection of different exercises for you to try. Some of these exercises take just a couple of minutes. None of these provide long-term solutions to anxiety, pressure or stress, but each can give you short bursts of respite.

Any action you take to reduce your stress level will provide some physical, mental or emotional benefits. For your emotional wellbeing I recommend you try to build a couple of these into your daily schedule. Some of these exercises can be done at your desk, so there's no excuse.

4.1 1 Minute Meditation

Even if you don't want to become a regular meditator you can enjoy a little stress relief with this mini-meditation. This very quick meditation is for anyone who is in a hurry.

This exercise is too short to offer any long-term benefits. However, if you do it frequently it will help you to programme your brain to take regular breaks.

Time required: 1 minute

Instructions:

1. Stop what you are doing. Do nothing for 1 minute

2. Smile. This relaxes your face muscles

3. Allow your mind and body to stop and just relax (it's only for 1 minute)

4. Take a deep breath and slowly release it to a count of 3-5

5. Repeat this deep breathing for 1 minute. During this time try to stay focused on your breathing and not your stressors

6. Give your body a quick shake and then resume your activities

Note: You can do this exercise as often as you like. It isn't a long-term stress buster but it's an opportunity to stop for a minute.

4.2 3 Minute Breathing Exercise (Quick Body Scan)

This short exercise is a cross between the Deep Breathing Exercise and the Mindfulness Relaxation Technique. The great thing about this exercise is it only takes 3 minutes to complete. We can all spare 3 minutes, no matter how busy we are.

Time required: 3 minutes

Instructions:

1. Sit in a quiet place and close your eyes. Ask yourself "what thoughts are going through my mind right now? What feelings am I having? What sensations am I experiencing?" Spend 1 minute thinking about these three questions

2. Now direct your attention to your breathing for 1 minute. Is your breathing deep or shallow? Just observe your breathing during this minute. If your mind starts to wander gently bring your focus back to your breathing

3. Now expand your awareness to take in your body as a whole. Notice if you feel any discomfort, pain or tension in any particular part of your body. If you do, imagine your breath soothing this discomfort or tension away and leaving your relaxed. Do this for 1 minute

4. When you feel ready slowly open your eyes. You are now ready to return to the activity you were doing before you took this short stress break

4.3 20 Minutes Hard Work

The best way to carry out any work is with complete mindfulness. By focusing on the task 100% you will find it less stressful, as you won't be allowing other thoughts to bog you down. This exercise works particularly well if you have an onerous task to complete.

Over time you can increase your work periods, but initially 20 minutes focused working is a great way to get things done.

Time required: 20 minutes

Instructions:

1. Before you start the task, promise yourself that for the next 20 minutes you will focus on this task and nothing else. This is a way of giving your mind permission to forget your worries for 20 minutes

2. Close your eyes for a moment and take a deep breath. Tell yourself "I am going to give my complete attention to [say the task] for 20 minutes. Then I'm going to have a short break"

3. Work for 20 minutes on this task and nothing else. Take a short break. This can be a physical break or just a change of activity'

4. Repeat steps 2 and 3 until the task is complete. Giving yourself short bursts of hard work will make you more focused and productive. Notice how your productivity improves

5. As you retrain your brain you will be able to do longer periods between breaks, or not use this exercise at all

4.4 Anger/Tension Release Exercise

As the name suggests, this is a quick exercise for releasing anger or tension. It's better for everyone if you take your anger and frustration out on a cushion rather than another person.

This exercise is designed to be less than 5 minutes, but you can make it a longer exercise if you want to. You need a cushion and a little space for this exercise as you are going to throw the cushion on the floor.

Time required: less than 5 minutes

1. Get a cushion. Stand up, close your eyes and breathe in as deeply as you possibly can

2. Breathe out slowly and loudly. Repeat steps 1 and 2 a couple of times or until you feel comfortable with deep breathing. Note: Some people take a few moments to adjust to this type of breathing

3. As you breathe in deeply this time, imagine transferring your anger and frustration to the cushion

4. Breathe out slowly and loudly. As soon as you have finished exhaling throw the cushion on the floor

5. Repeat steps 3 and 4 at least twice more

6. Now stop and notice how you're feeling. If you feel calmer move onto step 7. If not, keep repeating steps 3 and 4 until you feel calmer

7. Breathe in deeply once more and breathe out as slowly as you can. Shake your hands and wrists to shake off any remaining negative energy

8. Open your eyes and just stand for 1 minute (without speaking)

9. When you feel ready go back to what you were doing

4.5 Arms And Hands Deskercises

Deskercise is a catchy name given to exercises that you can do at your desk. There are lots of different versions of deskercises available. These exercises are based on the deskercises created by author, Emily Milam. Each of these exercises is designed for the workplace, and takes just a few minutes.

We already know that physical exercise is beneficial in tackling stress. Research suggests that even deskercise can be beneficial to physical health and mental wellbeing. A short burst of deskercise will have some benefit if you're stressed as it will provide a welcome distraction for a few minutes.

Time required: 2-5 minutes per exercise

Instructions:

This set of deskercises focuses on your arms and hands. You can do just one, some, or all eight of these exercises; the choice is yours.

The Triceps Exercise:
This exercise can be done anywhere as long as you have a sturdy desk and a chair without wheels. Sit at the very edge of your chair and place your hands on either side of your body while gripping the chair's edge.

With your feet planted on the floor a step or two away from the desk or chair, straighten up your arms to lift up your body. Next, bend your arms to reach a 90 degree angle so that your body dips down. Hold and re-straighten while keeping your body raised above the chair.

Repeat this exercise as often as you feel able to. If you find this exercise too difficult don't do it as there is nothing to be gained from injuring yourself.

The Namaste (Prayer Hands):
Sit upright in your chair with your feet flat on the floor. Next, bring your palms together in front of your chest and push both hands together powerfully until you feel your arm muscles contract. Hold your hands in prayer, pushed together, for 20 seconds. Release and repeat this exercise 10 times.

Give Yourself A Handshake:
Sit upright in your chair with your feet flat on the floor. Next, clasp your hands together as if giving yourself a handshake. Note: One thumb will be facing downwards and one thumb will be facing upwards.

With your right hand gently pull your left hand. Hold this position for 10 seconds and then release your hand. Now repeat the exercise with your left hand doing the pulling. Repeat this exercise 10 times per hand.

This exercise is designed to relax your hand and wrist muscles. This is a good exercise for anyone who spends long periods of time using a computer.

Punch The Air:
Ball each hand into a fist. Choose which hand you wish to start with. Using your fist, punch into the air like a champion. Do this exercise for one minute. As you do it, imagine the stress flying through the ceiling with each punch. Now switch arms and repeat the exercise.

Note: If it's a particular person causing you stress you can imagine him/her flying through the ceiling.

The Boxing Jab:
Stand (if you can). Throw out a few boxing jabs, hooks, and uppercuts in rapid succession (like you see boxers doing in the ring). Continue for a minute or longer to blow off steam and tone your arms, chest, and core muscles.

This is a great energiser if you're feeling sluggish. It's also a great way to release tension, pressure or stress. You could imagine punching your stressful situation or the person causing your stress.

Your Perfect Penguin Impression:
You might feel a little silly doing this exercise, but remember laughter is a great stress buster so just laugh at yourself.

Here's an opportunity to do your best penguin impression. Stand with your feel slightly apart and your arms by your sides (with your palms facing away from you). Push both arms backwards and hold to a count of 5. Slowly bring your arms back to your sides. Repeat this exercise 15 times.

For best results, keep your arms straight and stretched as long as possible. When you feel ready return to your previous activity.

The Mad Axe Man/Woman:
Stand with your feet slightly apart and clasp your hands together in front of you. Rest your clasped hands on your right shoulder as if holding an axe. Gently swing your imaginary axe by straightening your elbows and moving your hands toward your left thigh.

Next, bring your clasped hands to your left shoulder followed by a swing to right thigh. Repeat this exercise 10 times on each side. As you do this exercise imagine getting rid of the things causing you stress. See your axe breaking up the stress.

Imaginary Dumbbells:
For this exercise you need a bottle of water or a heavy stapler. This exercise can be done seated or standing. Take your imaginary dumbbell (bottle of water or stapler) in one hand with the palm facing upwards.

Starting at your thighs, bend your elbow and curl your arm up towards your chest. This is just like a regular dumbbell bicep curl. Hold this position to a count of 5 and then slowly lower your dumbbell back down.

Repeat this exercise 10 times and then switch arms. This deskercise is great if you're feeling anxious or stressed. It requires concentration and is a physical activity. This provides a short distraction from the things that are causing you anxiety.

4.6 Autogenic Training Relaxation Exercise

Autogenic training is a method of self-hypnosis. This was developed by German psychiatrist Johannes Heinrich Schultz, and was first published in 1932.

The autogenic training relaxation technique involves daily exercises that enable you to gain a state of relaxation through visualisation. Each practice session normally lasts around 15 minutes.

Autogenic training can be done lying down or sitting. Initially you might find it helpful for someone to read the instructions as you do this exercise.

Autogenic training normally takes 2-3 months to master. Practitioners claim it induces a sense of wellbeing, improves coping abilities and aids muscular relaxation. All of these are believed to play a part in stress management.

Devotees of autogenic relaxation say the results are worth the effort.

Time required: 15 minutes (per session)

Instructions:

1. Find a comfortable place to lie down or sit, and close your eyes

2. Breathe in deeply. Hold your breath for a count of 3-5 and then slowly exhale

3. Say "I am beginning to feel quiet now and I am beginning to feel relaxed". You can say this mantra out loud or silently; the choice is yours

4. Once you start to feel relaxed you're ready to begin the exercise. Continue taking slow regular breaths throughout the exercise

5. Focus on your right hand. Feel the skin on your palm becoming warm and relaxed. Notice the warmth in each finger and then feel this warmth spreading to the back of your right hand and wrist. Say "my hands feel heavy"

6. Now focus on your right forearm. Notice your right arm starting to feel heavy and relaxed

7. Repeat steps 5, 6 and 7 on your left hand and arm

8. Now focus on the tops of both arms and your shoulders. Say "my arms and shoulders feel heavy". Notice your arms/shoulders becoming warm and heavy

9. Next, turn your attention to your legs. Feel your legs becoming warm. Feel this warmth spreading all the way down each leg to your ankles and feet. Feel your legs and feet becoming heaving and relaxed. Say "my feet, ankles, knees and hips feel heavy"

10. When you're ready, move your focus to your head. Imagine a warm breeze blowing across your face. Notice your face and head relaxing, and feel your eyelids getting heavy

11. Notice your jaw and neck feeling heavy but relaxed. Say "my neck and jaw feel heavy"

12. Now imagine the sun shining down on you. Feel the warmth on the front of your body. Notice your chest and stomach relaxing in this lovely warmth

13. Say "my heart is calm and regular. My breathing is calm and regular. My solar plexus is calm and regular"

14. Notice that your entire body is now relaxed. Feel it becoming warm and calm. Say "my whole body feels quiet, comfortable and deeply relaxed"

15. Once your mind is quiet and your body feels comfortable and deeply relaxed visualise one of the following images:
- A sandy beach with the waves gently lapping on the shore
- A cool, clear stream gently trickling over pebbles and weaving its way towards its destination
- A waterfall (e.g. Niagara Falls)
- A fluffy cloud drifting across the sky
- A camp fire with flames dancing and making images

It doesn't matter which one you choose. Your intuition will choose the right one for you.

16. Focus on this image for a few minutes. Enjoy this sense of deep relaxation for a few minutes

17. When you're ready, slowly bring your attention back to the present, but don't open your eyes yet. Notice the room around you, notice the surface you're sitting or lying on, hear any sounds around you

18. Start to reawaken your body by wiggling your fingers and toes. Now shake your arms and move your legs. Finally have a good stretch (like a cat does when it wakes up)

19. When you're ready open your eyes and become fully alert again. Allow yourself at least 1 minute before you speak or resume your activity.

4.7 Body Awareness Relaxation Exercise

Body awareness is one of the major foundations from which children develop good movement skills. This exercise is similar to, but not the same as, the Autogenic Training Relaxation Exercise.

In our fast-paced society we push our minds and bodies to the limit. This is often at the expense of our physical and mental wellbeing. Body awareness (sometimes referred to as body scan) simply uses relaxation to focus on the sensations in each part of your body.

You don't need any specialist equipment for this exercise but you do need to be able to lie down.

Time required: 30 minutes

Instructions:

1. Lie on your back, legs uncrossed, arms straight at your sides and your eyes open or closed. Initially you may find it easier to do this exercise with your eyes closed. Over time you will be able to do this with your eyes open

2. Breathe in deeply through your nose. Hold your breath for a count of 3-5 and then exhale very slowly through your mouth

3. Repeat this breathing exercise for a couple of minutes until you feel relaxed

4. When you're ready to start, shift your attention to the toes of your right foot. Take a moment to focus on how your toes feel

5. Notice any sensations you feel in your toes while continuing to also focus on your breathing. Imagine each deep breath flowing straight down to your toes. Repeat this exercise for 1 minute - all the time remaining focused on this area only

6. Move your focus to the sole of your right foot. Notice any sensations you feel in this part of your body. Imagine each breath flowing straight to the sole of your foot. Repeat this exercise for 1 minute - all the time remaining focused on this area

7. Move your focus to your right ankle. Notice any sensations you feel in your ankle and imagine each breath flowing straight to your ankle. Repeat this exercise for 1 minute - all the time remaining focused on this area

8. Repeat this exercise for your right calf, knee, thigh and hip

9. Now switch to your left side. Repeat steps 4-8 on your left side, finishing with your left hip

10. Next, move up your torso. Start with your lower back. Continue to breathe deeply and feel each breath going to your lower back. Take a minute or two to focus on the way it feels

11. Now move onto your abdomen. As you breathe deeply sense your breath reaching your abdomen. Be aware of how it feels. Spend 1 minute focusing on any sensations you feel in your abdomen

12. When you're ready, move to your upper back. Imagine each deep breath flowing straight to your upper back and releasing the tension. Focus on the way your upper back feels for 1 minute

13. As you continue to breathe deeply, focus your attention on your chest. Imagine each deep breath flowing to your chest. Focus on the way your chest feels for 1 minute

14. Now move onto your shoulders. You might like to spend a little longer on your shoulders as this is an area that absorbs a lot of tension. As you breathe deeply sense each breath spreading across your shoulders and soothing away any tension. Spend as long as necessary focusing on any sensations you feel in your shoulders and imagine the tension disappearing

15. Next, imagine each deep breath flowing to your fingers on your right hand. Repeat this exercise for 1 minute - all the time remaining focused on your fingers

16. Move your focus to your right hand, moving up to your wrist. Notice any sensations you feel in your hand as each breath flows to your right hand and wrist. Repeat this exercise for 1 minute - all the time remaining focused on this area

17. Move your focus to your right forearm, elbow and upper arm until you reach your shoulder. Notice any sensations you feel in your arm and imagine each breath flowing through your right arm. Repeat this exercise for 1 minute - all the time remaining focused on your arm

18. Now switch to your left side. Repeat steps 15-17 on your left side, finishing at the top of your left arm

19. Next, move through your neck and throat. Imagine your deep breathing soothing these areas and taking all the tension away. Repeat this for 1 minute (or longer if needed)

20. Finally move onto your face and the back and top of your head. Pay close attention to your jaw, chin, lips, tongue, nose, cheeks, eyes, forehead, temples and scalp. Imagine each deep breath covering your face and head, and soothing away tension. Repeat this for 1 minute

21. When you reach the very top of your head, let your breath reach out beyond your body and imagine yourself hovering above your physical body. Repeat this for 1 minute

22. After completing the body awareness relaxation exercise, relax for a few minutes in silence and stillness. While you're doing this notice how your body feels. If you notice any areas of tension you might like to work on it again. When you're ready open your eyes slowly

Note: As you work through each part of your body pay close attention to any area that causes you pain or discomfort.

If you notice any painful or uncomfortable areas spend a little longer on them. Simply keep taking deep breaths and see the energy flowing to that part of the body and releasing the tension. If the pain persists consult your GP.

4.8 Cardiovascular Deskercises

Deskercise is a catchy name given to exercises that you can do at your desk. There are lots of different versions of deskercises available. These exercises are based on the deskercises created by author, Emily Milam. Each of these exercises is designed for the workplace, and takes just a few minutes.

We already know that physical exercise is beneficial in tackling stress. Research suggests that even deskercise can be beneficial to physical health and mental wellbeing. A short burst of deskercise will have some benefit if you're stressed as it will provide a welcome distraction for a few minutes.

Time required: 2-5 minutes per exercise

Instructions:

You can do just one, some, or all of these six exercises; the choice is yours.

The Twinkle Toes:
Emily suggests tapping into your inner Fred Astaire. Speedily tap your toes on the floor under your desk for 2 minutes. This isn't a major stress reliever, but it does provide a temporary distraction.

Distraction often helps to get things into perspective, so indulge yourself.

The Stair Master:
Look for every opportunity to take the stairs instead of the lift or escalator. If you really want to give your legs a workout take two stairs at a time. Initially you may feel this stretching your leg muscles.

You will feel more energised if you do this regularly. Feeling energised means you have a more positive reaction to stressful situations. It also provides you with better coping skills when stress hits.

The Slog, The Jog:
Stress is an energy sapper and so is slogging away at your desk for hours. Re-energising yourself will make you more productive and give you better coping skills.

You might feel silly doing this exercise. If so, why not try to get your colleagues to do it with you.

Take a mini break for a stationary jog. Simply stand up and jog where you're standing. If you're willing to push yourself a little more, raise your knees. Do this repeatedly for 2 minutes.

While you're doing this imagine jogging on your stressful situations. Each time your foot touches the floor you're flattening the things (or people) who have been putting you under pressure.

The Celebratory Split Squat Jumps:
With feet hip-width apart, step your left leg back two feet and balance on the ball of your foot. Next, lower into a lunge. Then switch feet so that your left foot is planted firmly in front and your right leg is now behind. Repeat 10-12 times on each side.

Each time you lower your foot into a lunge imagine one of your stressors being released. If you only have one stressful situation, during this exercise repeatedly focus on getting rid of it.

Walk Around The Office:
Instead of sending an email or picking up the phone to speak to someone in your office, go and see them. This will give you a mini break from your desk, which is necessary to maintain optimum performance when you're working.

Regular breaks are essential to mental wellbeing as they give your brain a short rest. This in turn, helps with developing a positive attitude to stressful situations. Short breaks also encourage clear thinking.

The Mover And Shaker:
Release stress and spark some energy with a quick bout of seated dancing when no one is looking! This will help release the feel good chemical (Serotonin). As I've said before, a positive attitude really helps with stress management.

4.9 Caribbean Beach Guided Meditation

Ideally you want to find someone with a soothing voice to lead you through this guided meditation. Alternatively, read the instructions and visualise the Caribbean beach sequence described below.

This meditation takes approximately 20 minutes, but at the end of it you won't feel as if it was that long. This is a very lovely stress release technique that's guaranteed to make you feel better for a while.

Time required: 20 minutes

Instructions:

1. Sit comfortably in your seat and allow your shoulders to drop. Alternatively, lie down

2. Close your eyes. You're always in control so you can return to your awakened state at any time by simply opening your eyes

3. Now get rid of any preconceived ideas you have about meditation and just approach this with an open mind. The worst thing that will happen is you'll think it's boring or not for me. Hopefully you will enjoy the experience and feel relaxed at the end of it

4. Take a deep breath. Try to breathe right down to your stomach. You may find it hard to breathe this deeply to start with but just stick with it

5. Now exhale (breathe out) very slowly

6. Repeat this deep breathing 5 times

7. Breathe in deeply and exhale once more. As you breathe out this time feel your arms, legs and body become relaxed. Know that you are perfectly safe and in control. You can open your eyes at any time

8. Continue to breathe in deeply and exhale slowly

9. Each time you exhale let go of your thoughts. Whatever thought comes into your mind, just allow it to drift away. If you can't let go of a particular thought make a mental note to deal with it later

10. Continue breathing in and out, and as you do so feel your mind and body relax

11. Notice the sense of peace, tranquillity and contentment you're feeling right now. All your thoughts and worries are gone for a little while. Know this is your relaxation time

12. Now imagine yourself on a Caribbean Island, having a very relaxing holiday

13. See yourself walking along a beautiful creamy-white beach. Feel the warm sand under your feet and the sun beating down on you, warming and relaxing your body

14. Now look to the sky. All you can see is a clear blue sky with the occasional white fluffy cloud drifting by. Notice how the clouds are drifting by without a care in the world. These clouds represent you right now. You don't have a care in the world - all your problems are a long way away

15. Now look at the crystal clear sea. It's somewhere between blue and aqua in colour. Notice how soothing it feels. Feel the water washing your cares and worries away

16. You notice a small rowing boat on the shoreline. This boat is waiting to collect your worries and take them away. With each step you take along the beach release one of your worries, concerns or issues. Imagine each one being deposited into this little boat

17. Keep walking until you've loaded all your worries into the boat. Now see someone pushing the boat out to sea. Notice how you feel as if a load has been lifted from your shoulders

18. Watch the waves take the boat further and further out to sea. Soon it's completely out of sight and with it your worries

19. Now it's time for a little me-time so you slowly head back towards the beach bar. As you walk you become much more aware of your beautiful surroundings. Notice the colour of the sea, the sky, the sand, palm trees, and anything else you see, smell or feel

20. As you get near the beach bar the barman gives you a wave and immediately starts to prepare your favourite cocktail

21. Your beach bar is typically Caribbean - made out of driftwood and straw. As you get closer to the bar you hear a steel band playing

22. Your sun lounger is already waiting for you, nestled between the pool and the palm trees

23. As you settle down the barman appears with your cocktail, beautifully decorated with exotic fruits. It's been lovingly made just for you

24. As you lie there relaxing you suddenly become more sensitive to your surroundings. You hear the gentle rustle of the palm trees. You hear a 'plop' as a coconut falls from the tree into the sand. You hear

the waves gently lapping against the shoreline, and in the distance you hear music and laughter

25. This is your very special and private place in the Caribbean and you can come back here any time you like. No one and nothing is going to disturb you here as this is your private place

26. Before we leave this special place take a moment to look around. Notice how you feel right now - the peace and tranquillity is just what you needed today. Your body and mind needed this time to relax and be peaceful. Notice how much lighter you feel

27. Take one last look at your surroundings and commit it all to memory. Know you can come back here whenever you want to

28. We're going to have to say goodbye to the Caribbean now

29. When you're ready bring yourself back into the room. Feel yourself sitting in the chair. Slowly open your eyes. There's no rush; take as long as you like

30. Don't say anything, just give yourself a minute to readjust and notice how wonderfully relaxed you feel

4.10 Central Channel Meditation Exercise

This meditation focuses on a beam of energy instead of your breath. As you breathe in you draw a beam of energy in through the top of your head. As you breathe out you release this beam of energy through the same place on the top of your head.

Time required: 20-40 minutes

Instructions:

1. Sit comfortably. Close your eyes

2. Take a deep breath and bend forward slowly. Breathe out loudly through your mouth

3. Repeat this breathing exercise 3 times

4. Now sit still and breathe naturally. Notice you abdomen expand and contract with each in/out breath

5. Don't focus on your breath. Instead focus on the beam of energy entering the crown of your head through the 'medicine palace'. This is a point two inches above your hairline

6. Feel this beam of energy flowing in through this point each time you breathe in. Follow this beam of energy down through your chakras to the sacral chakra (two inches below your navel)

7. See this beam of energy flowing back up through your chakras. Breathe it out through the medicine palace

8. Repeat this for 20-40 minutes. To get the optimum benefit from this type of meditation it should be done once or twice daily

Note: You may notice a sensation as the energy flows in and out of the medicine palace. You may experience feelings of warmth, tingling or numbness. This is perfectly natural and nothing to worry about.

4.11 Centring Technique Exercise

Centring is a technique that originated, and is still used, in Aikido. Everything, including stress, is energy. The centring process helps to manage energy. This is why it's good for stress management.

To be able to master the art of centring you have to be able to do deep breathing. If you're not familiar with deep breathing refer to the Deep Breathing Exercise. Concentration and imagination are also important to the success of this technique.

Time required: 20-60 minutes

Instructions:

1. Sit down in a chair. Get into a comfortable position where your spine is fairly straight and your feet are on the floor. Place one hand on your chest and the other on your stomach

2. Close your eyes. Breathe in deeply, through your nose. The hand on your stomach should rise, but the hand on your chest should move very little

3. Slowly exhale (breathe out)

4. Keep repeating this deep breathing until your focus is only on your breathing and nothing else. This will come with practice. Initially your mind might be flooded with thoughts. This is normal

5. Now, locate your physical centre of gravity (your solar plexus). This is a little below your waist and above your belly button. This is the part of your body that grounds and stabilises you

6. Once you've found this energy centre breathe in deeply and exhale slowly. Repeat this 5 times

7. From now on, you're going to see your breath travelling through your upper body and solar plexus. See each in-breath going down your spine and legs to your toes

8. As your breath reaches your feet imagine roots pushing down through the floor and into the soil below. Feel the rich earth and notice how healthy it is

9. Imagine your breath continuing its journey. Feel it pushing down through the waters under the soil, through the bedrock, and into the centre of the earth

10. Do you have any tension or fear left? If so, release it through your 'roots' and deep into the centre of the earth. Imagine a fire at the centre of the earth. See yourself throwing all your stress and negative feelings into the fire

11. Now draw some of that fire up into your body. Feel the fire as the earth's living creative energy. Bring it up through the rock, the water and the soil. Bring the fire into your legs and feet, like a tree's roots drawing up water and nutrients

12. Bring this fire energy up your spine. Imagine your spine growing like a tree trunk, reaching up to the sky. Feel the fire making you strong. Bring the fire into your heart, and any other part of your body that needs healing right now

13. Imagine this fire energy flowing into you. Straighten your back and re-focus on your breath. Feel this fire renewing your energy

14. Now, direct the energy up through your arms and out of your hands. Feel it move up through your neck, throat and face, and out the top of your head. Visualise branches of energy that reach up to the sky. Let these branches spread around you and reach back down to touch the earth. These branches are forming a protective web around you

15. Take a moment to look at your web of energy. Are there any places that need to be repaired or strengthened? If so, send energy in that direction

16. Now, imagine the energy of the sun, shining down on your leaves and branches. Feel the sun's heat warming and soothing you. Notice how relaxed you feel now

17. Repeat steps 7-16 as many times as you want or need to

18. When you're ready, come back to stillness. As you breathe deeply, notice where in your body this grounded place lives. Touch that place. Choose an image or phrase for your grounded state. This will be your anchor to help you ground quickly in any situation, in future

19. Slowly open your eyes and look around you. Notice how you feel now. For example, are you relaxed or more aware of your body and mental wellbeing? Are you still stressed?

You may like to repeat a mantra as you're doing this centring exercise. If so, repeat the following mantra to yourself "every day in every way I am getting better and better".

Next time you're feeling stressed focus on your anchor (as per step 18). If this doesn't help calm you then you may need to repeat the entire centring technique exercise.

4.12 Chakra Meditation

Chakras are the energy centres positioned vertically throughout your body. Each is responsible for controlling the flow and distribution of energy in your body. If your chakras are balanced you will feel physically, mentally and emotionally much better.

Meditating with chakras requires a leap of faith. The idea of this meditation is to release blocked energy. You don't want energy whizzing around your system too fast as this is not grounding or soothing.

Note: When visualising your chakras you may not see them as perfect circles. They may look a little rough or wobbly. This is fine, just work with what you see and allow your mind to heal them.

You will find information about chakras is chapter three.

Time required: 20-40 minutes

Instructions:

1. You can do this meditation lying or sitting down, whichever you prefer. Breathe in deeply, hold your breath to a count of 3-5 and then slowly breathe out

2. Repeat this until you start to feel relaxed

3. When you're ready visualise a beam of white light entering through your crown chakra (top of your head)

4. See this white light flowing down to your root chakra (at the base of your spine)

5. Imagine your root chakra as a bright red orb. See it spinning freely. Don't worry if you can't see it as the perfect shade of red. It may appear as maroon or any other shade of red

6. Continue breathing deeply and slowly. Take each breath down to this chakra

7. Repeat this until you feel ready to move onto the next chakra. Your intuition will tell you when you're ready to move on

8. With your next in-breath see this beam of white light going down to your sacral chakra. The sacral chakra is two inches below your navel

9. Imagine your sacral chakra as an orange orb. See it spinning freely

10. Repeat steps 6 and 7

11. Repeat these steps for each chakra in turn. The order is solar plexus chakra (yellow), heart chakra (green or pink), throat chakra (blue) and third eye chakra (indigo)

12. Finally you reach your crown chakra (violet in colour). See your crown chakra spinning freely with beautiful violet energy

13. Once you have finished visualising your crown chakra, see all your chakras spinning at once

14. Now visualise your beam of white light flowing down like a mountain waterfall. See it going through your crown chakra and right down through your body to your feet. See it going deep into the ground beneath you

15. If you have any remaining negative energy, let it go. Release any negative energy through your root chakra. As you release negative energy see new positive energy coming in through your crown chakra

16. Notice that your body now feels natural and balanced. Take a final deep breath and see this white light flowing freely through your entire body

17. When you feel ready, slowly open your eyes. Don't say or do anything for at least 1 minute. Just allow yourself to be still

18. When you feel completely grounded resume your activities

4.13 Chi Visualisation Exercise

Chi is the term for universal energy, or the energy that surrounds us and everything around us. Chi is the energy that gives us life because it fuels every single process in our bodies.

In order for your body to function at its optimum level energy needs to be able to flow freely. Tension and stress stop this free flow of energy.

When you are worried or stressed, you send frequencies of fear and insecurity through your body. Imagine this as energy shockwaves.

The natural reaction of your body is to protect itself by tensing the muscles that are related to self-protection. Your neck, back and shoulder muscles are the first to react to this shockwave.

When your chi energy is flowing freely it enhances your creativity at all levels, including - art, business/work, relationships, etc.

Time required: 5-30 minutes

Instructions:

1. Lie down or sit in a chair if that feels more comfortable. Get into a comfortable position where your spine is fairly straight. If you're lying down rest your arms by your sides. If you're sitting in a chair place your feet on the floor and your hands in your lap

2. Breathe in deeply through your nose. Hold your breath up to a count of 3-5 and then slowly exhale through your mouth. Keep repeating this deep breathing until you start to feel relaxed

3. Next, imagine a bowl filled with warm oil nestling in your pelvis (this represents your chi energy). You can imagine it's your favourite aromatherapy oil if this helps with your visualisation

4. With each in-breath picture the oil rising up through your spine. See it going all the way up to the top of your head

5. As you slowly breathe out, see the oil flowing down your front and trickling back into the bowl

6. Repeat this exercise for at least 5 minutes, or until you feel completely relaxed. If you spend a few minutes doing this exercise every day you will notice a change in your energy

Note: Chi energy is the way Reiki healers treat illnesses.

4.14 Cloud 9 Meditation

This particular meditation exercise is designed for when you're in an aeroplane. I realise that you may not be flying anywhere when you read this book. I have chosen to include this exercise as you may wish to use it next time you travel.

Some people find air travel a stressful experience so I hope this might help restore a little calm.

Time required: As long as you wish

Instructions:

1. Make sure you are sitting comfortably before you start. Loosen your clothes and remove your shoes. Put your feet on the foot rest or on a pillow

2. Relax, breathe gently and close your eyes

3. Lean your head on the backrest and drop your shoulders

4. As you inhale imagine a pale translucent light pouring in through your third eye chakra (centre of your forehead). See this light filling your body

5. As you exhale, imagine darkness flushing out of your body. Imagine this darkness leaving through your bottom

6. Keep repeating this until you feel all the darkness has left you. Imagine your body is now filled with beautiful light energy

7. Now imagine that the plane is no longer surrounding you. Instead you are floating on your own cloud or floating in the clear blue sky. If you prefer you can imagine a lovely night sky filled with stars

8. Feel the air supporting you and the wind caressing your temples

9. When you're ready end your meditation

4.15 Core Deskercises

Deskercise is a catchy name given to exercises that you can do at your desk. There are lots of different versions of deskercises available. These exercises are based on the deskercises created by author, Emily Milam. Each of these exercises is designed for the workplace, and takes just a few minutes.

We already know that physical exercise is beneficial in tackling stress. Research suggests that even deskercise can be beneficial to physical health and mental wellbeing. A short burst of deskercise will have some benefit if you're stressed as it will provide a welcome distraction for a few minutes.

Time required: 2–5 minutes per exercise

Instructions:

This set of exercises focuses on your core muscles. You can do just one or all three of these exercises; the choice is yours.

The Desk Chair Swivel:
Sit upright in your chair with the feet hovering off the floor. Hold the edge of your desk with your fingers and thumb. Use your core muscles to swivel the chair from side to side. Don't use your arms to move you. Repeat this exercise 15 times.

If it helps, think about the person or situation that is causing your stress. This will help give you the strength you need. With each twist imagine you are pushing the person or situation away from you.

The Fab Abs Squeeze:
This is a silent deskercise that can be done covertly. Take a deep breath and tighten your abdominal muscles, bringing them in towards the spin. Stay squeezed up to a count of 5. Slowly exhale.

Repeat this exercise 10 times, or as many times as you feel comfortable doing. Each time you exhale, imagine the stress leaving you.

You may like to do this exercise every time you start to feel anxious.

The Chair Wheelie:
You need a chair with wheels for this exercise. While seated in your chair position yourself at arm's length from your desk. Grasp the edge of the desk with both hands.

Next, engage your core muscles. Raise your feet slightly off the ground. Using your arms pull the chair forward until your chest touches the desk's edge. Roll back by pushing yourself away from the desk, with your feet still raised. Repeat this exercise 20 times.

As you need to concentrate on what you are doing, this exercise provides a temporary distraction from your stressors.

4.16 Deep Breathing Exercise

Have you ever noticed your breathing when you're relaxed? Next time you feel relaxed; take a moment to notice how your body and mind feels.

Deep breathing exercises can help you relax, because they make your body feel like it does when you are already relaxed. Five minutes 'time out' can be calming and refreshing, without the need to make any big changes to your life.

Deep breathing is one of the best ways to lower stress in your body. This is because when you breathe deeply it sends a message to your brain to calm down and relax. The brain then sends this message to your body.

When you are stressed you will have an increased heart rate and faster breathing. You may also have high blood pressure. As you learn to breathe deeply and relax these will decrease.

You can do this exercise wherever you are, and can spend as little or as much time as you wish. To do this exercise, all you need is a chair. I recommend you build this exercise into your daily routine several times a day.

This deep breathing exercise is helpful if you have trouble getting to sleep. Get into bed, relax and start deep breathing until you drift off to sleep.

Time required: 2-30 minutes

Instructions:

1. Sit down in a chair. Get into a comfortable position where your spine is fairly straight and your feet are on the floor. Place one hand on your chest and the other on your stomach

2. Breathe in deeply, through your nose. The hand on your stomach should rise, but the hand on your chest should move very little

3. Slowly exhale (breathe out) until your lungs are empty

4. Keep repeating this deep breathing until you notice your breathing becomes slower and deeper

5. Now you've got the hang of this we're going to increase the effectiveness of your deep breathing. Breathe in deeply through your nose again. This time try to hold your breath to a count of 3-5 before breathing out. This might not be possible to start with

Exhale slowly, through your mouth. Push out as much air as you can while contracting your abdominal muscles. The hand on your stomach should move in as you exhale, but your other hand should move very little

6. Take another deep in-breath. Imagine that your body is feeling very relaxed. Imagine this feeling flowing through every part of your body. As you breathe out, imagine all the stress leaving you. After a few minutes you should start to feel more peaceful and relaxed

7. If you're doing this exercise with a group, stop talking for a few minutes. Allow each person to relax as fully as possible. Do this exercise for 5-30 minutes, depending upon the time you have available and how long you wish to spend

If you're concerned that this exercise will put you to sleep, keep your practice to just 5 minutes. On the other hand, if you're having trouble sleeping, this exercise may be very helpful. It helps to still the mind and so makes it easier to go to sleep.

4.17 Empty Mind Meditation

As the name suggests, this type of meditation requires you to empty all thoughts from your mind. The idea is visualise air passing through your mind and just relax in this empty space. This allows peacefulness to take over and induces a state of deep relaxation.

Time required: 20 minutes

Instructions:

1. Close your eyes. Breathe in deeply and slowly exhale
2. Repeat this deep breathing until you start to relax
3. Now as you breathe in visualise the element of air passing through your mind. This helps to dissolve your thoughts. If thoughts pop into your mind acknowledge them and then see the air blowing them away
4. Continue this deep breathing and see the air passing through your mind
5. As your meditation becomes deeper see the air brushing the inside of your skull as it passes through your mind. Try to remain in this empty mind state for as long as possible
6. Keep repeating this breathing and empty mind sensation for at least 20 minutes
7. When you're ready slowly open your eyes. Just sit quietly for at least 1 minute
8. Resume your activities when you're ready

4.18 Focused Meditation

This type of meditation focuses on something, and is done with your eyes open. You can focus on music, an object, a mantra or a single thought. Most commonly people focus on an ornament or candle flame during this meditation.

You might like to burn some incense while you do this meditation. Many people find the smell of incense helps them to relax.

Time required: 15-20 minutes

Instructions:

1. Choose a target for your focus

2. Get into a comfortable sitting position. Breathe deeply a few times to help your mind and body to relax

3. Start to focus on your chosen target. Notice all the sensations you feel while focusing on this e.g. sounds, smells, images etc. Just focus your attention on this and nothing else

4. If your mind starts to wander, acknowledge the thought and then return to your object. The more you do this the easier it gets

5. Ideally you are aiming to do this exercise for 15-20 minutes, but even a few minutes will be beneficial

4.19 Freeze Relaxation Exercise

Taking regular moments of rest makes us more efficient. This quick exercise is called 'freeze relaxation' as you literally stop what you're doing for 2 minutes. You can do this anywhere and at any time. More importantly, you don't need any equipment to do this exercise.

This exercise is taken from Eric Harrison's Teach Yourself to Meditate book.

Time required: 2 minutes

Instructions:

1. Whatever you're doing, tell yourself to 'freeze'

2. Hold your posture exactly as it is, but carry on breathing normally

3. Do a quick body scan from head to toe. As you do this make a mental note of any areas of tension in your body

4. Now, become aware of your breathing

5. When you feel in tune with your breathing, say 'defrost' and allow the tension to release

6. Make little adjustments as appropriate e.g. sit or stand straighter. You may need to loosen your shoulders or neck muscles. If your eyes are sore close them for a few seconds

7. Do another quick body scan to see if you still have any tension

8. Repeat this until you've tackled all the areas of tension in your body

9. Take a deep breath and sigh as you breathe out

10. Notice your mood changing

11. When you're ready, return to whatever you were doing

It's good to allow yourself to 'chill'; even for just a few minutes. Whenever you notice you are getting tense or stressed spend a couple of minutes doing this 'freeze relaxation exercise'.

4.20 Giving A Hand Massage

Giving someone a hand massage is something that can be done anywhere and at any time. It only takes a few minutes but this exercise is a great stress buster for the receiver. As the giver you may find it relaxing too.

Time required: 5 minutes

Instructions:

1. Coat your hands with a thin layer of lotion or hand cream. Rub the top and bottom of the other person's hands so you spread the lotion over their hands

2. Steps 2 and 3 are necessary to warm up the muscles for the massage.

Grasp the other person's left hand so that his/her palm is facing the floor. Put your thumbs on his/her wrist and your fingers around the underside of his/her hand. Gently pull outward and toward you, stretching the muscles as you pull. Gently lower their left hand

3. Grasp the other person's right hand so that his/her palm is facing the floor. Put your thumbs on his/her wrist and your fingers around the underside of his/her hand. Gently pull outward and toward you, stretching the muscles as you pull. Gently lower their right hand

4. Now start the massage. Gently rub your thumbs in small, circular motions across the back of his/her left hand. Start with the knuckles and progress toward the wrist. Include the wrist in the massage for better muscle relaxation. Gently lower their left hand

5. Take their right hand and repeat step 4. Gently lower their right hand

6. Place both thumbs on the other person's left wrist. With light but firm pressure, pull your thumbs down the hand. Move one thumb

between their pinkie and ring finger and the other thumb between the thumb and forefinger.

Place your thumbs back at the wrist and repeat the motion. This time push down into the spaces surrounding the middle finger. Gently lower their left hand.

7. Place both thumbs on their right wrist. Repeat step 6. Gently lower their right hand.

Note: This will stretch and relax the areas between the fingers

8. Turn their hands over so that the palms are facing up. Put your thumbs on his/her left wrist. Your fingers will be holding their palm. Gently pull outward and toward you, stretching the muscles as you pull. Gently lower their left hand

9. Put your thumbs on his/her right wrist and your fingers holding their palm. Repeat step 8. Gently lower their right hand

10. Starting with their left hand move your thumbs in small, circular strokes across the entire palm and up to the wrist. Pay special attention to the pad beneath the thumb, as the muscles there can get very tight. Gently lower their left hand

11. With their right repeat step 10. Gently lower their right hand

12. Turn their hands back over so the palms face the floor. Holding his/her left hand, place your thumb and forefinger on either side of the pinkie finger and squeeze. Use small squeezing movements to massage all the way up to the fingertip. When you reach the fingernail give the finger a light tug

13. Release the finger; place your thumb on top and your forefinger on the bottom of the pinkie finger. Use small squeezing movements to massage all the way up the finger. When you reach the fingernail, give the finger a light tug

14. Repeat steps 12 and 13 for each finger on his/her left hand. Gently lower their left hand

15. Now repeat steps 12, 13 and 14 on their right hand. Gently lower his/her right hand

Shake your hands and wrists to shake off any negative energy you picked up from the receiver

4.21 Hand Massage Self-treatment

If there isn't anyone available to give you a hand massage you can give yourself one. You can do this anywhere, at any time, and it only takes a few minutes.

Hand cream is optional for this exercise.

Time required: 5 minutes

Instructions:

1. Using your right thumb and forefinger gently pinch each fingertip and thumb on your left hand. The pressure applied to each fingertip should be firm, but not painful. Repeat each finger/thumb 3 times

2. With your left thumb and forefinger repeat step 1 on right hand

3. Using your right thumb and forefinger gently pinch the sides of your fingers on your left hand. Repeat this exercise 3 times per finger/thumb

4. Using your left thumb and forefinger repeat step 3

5. Using your right thumb vigorously rub the top and palm side of each finger on your left hand

6. Using your left thumb step 5 on your right hand

7. Using your right thumb and forefinger vigorously rub the sides of your fingers on your left hand

8. Using your left thumb and forefinger repeat step 7 on your right hand

9. This part of the exercise involves finger tugging. Grasp each finger and thumb in turn, at the base. Pull firmly, but not so hard that you pull your fingers out of their sockets. Start with your left hand and then repeat the exercise for your right hand. If it hurts, don't do it

10. Using your right thumb and forefinger gently pinch and pull the webbed areas between the fingers on your left hand. Take care as this may be painful

11. Using your left thumb and forefinger repeat step 10 on your right hand

12. Gently massage the top of your left hand with your right thumb or fingertips

13. Repeat step 12 on your right hand

14. With your right thumb gently massage your left inner wrist

15. Repeat step 14 on your right inner wrist

16. With your right thumb firmly massage the palm of your left hand

17. Repeat step 16 on your right hand

18. Using your right thumb centre yourself by pressing your thumb deeply in the centre of your left palm

19. Repeat step 18 on your right palm

This is one stress relief exercise that you can easily do while sitting in meetings

4.22 Heart Centred Meditation

This meditation works on your heart chakra to release any fears and sadness you are feeling. This is a variation on the visualisation exercise as you work with a ball of healing-love energy.

You can do this meditation sitting or lying down, whichever feels most comfortable for you.

Time required: 20-30 minutes

Instructions:

1. Sit or lie in a position that feels comfortable for you. If sitting you can sit on a chair or on the floor with your back against the wall. It really doesn't matter for this exercise

2. Take a deep breath and hold onto it. While holding your breathe tense as many muscles as you can

3. Slowly exhale and release your muscles. At the same time feel yourself releasing the tension

4. Repeat steps 2 and 3 twice more. You should now feel a little more relaxed. If not, keep repeating steps 2 and 3 until you feel some of the tension going

5. Visualise your muscles feeling relaxed and bathed in brilliant white light

6. Continue to breathe deeply and slowly. Starting at your toes and working up to your head, visualise each part of your body bathed in brilliant white light

7. Notice any discomfort in any part of your body as you do this. If you find any tension spend a little more time focusing on that part of your body

8. You should now be feeling relaxed. Draw your attention to your heart chakra (in your chest area)

9. Visualise a tiny ball of light resting in the centre of your chest. This ball of light can be any colour you choose

10. Keep breathing deeply and slowly. With each breath see your ball of light getting bigger. As this ball of light gets bigger feel yourself growing calmer and more peaceful

11. Allow your ball of light to grow as big as you feel comfortable with. This is the ball of healing loving energy, which will soothe away your fears and sadness

12. Allow your ball of light to travel wherever it is needed in your body. Don't try to control it, just be guided by your intuition. All you need to do is keep focusing on your ball of light as you breathe in and out

Note: Your ball of healing loving energy may stay in your heart chakra. This is fine; it just means your heart is the area that needs some peace and love

13. If you know anyone else who needs some nurturing, you can visualise yourself sending this healing loving energy to them

14. When you feel your meditation has finished slowly bring your attention back into the room. Feel yourself sitting or lying down and become aware of your surroundings once more

15. When you feel ready, slowly open your eyes. Allow yourself a minute before you speak or do anything. Just spend this time centring yourself

16. When you feel ready, resume your activities

4.23 How Stressed Are You? Exercise

Are you feeling stressed right now? Do you know how stressed you are? Complete this quick questionnaire to find out whether you're slightly under pressure, feeling full blown stress or somewhere in between.

Time required: 10 minutes

Instructions:

1. Tick each of the symptoms that you're currently experiencing

Physical Symptoms	✓	Emotional Symptoms	✓
Allergies		Anxiety	
Breathlessness		Becoming cynical	
Change of menstrual cycle		Decrease in self-confidence or self-esteem	
Chest pains or palpitations		Feeling angry	
Chest tightness		Feeling guilty	
Constipation or diarrhoea		Feelings of helplessness	
Frequent illnesses		Feeling tense	
General aches and pains		Feeling your life it out of control	
Headaches or migraines		Irritable or intolerant	
Indigestion or heartburn		Lack of concentration	
Muscle twitches or spams		Lack of enthusiasm or negative thinking	
Nausea		Mood swings	
Skin rashes or other skin conditions		Weepy/tearful	
Sleep problems			
Tiredness or fatigue			
Weight variation (up or down)			
Behavioural Symptoms	✓	**Psychological Symptoms/Negative Thoughts**	✓
Aggressive or passive behaviour		I can't cope	
Change of interest in sex		I don't know what to do	
Drinking or smoking more than usual		I don't seem to be able to get on top of anything	
Drop in performance at work		I feel helpless	
Increased use of drugs or medication (legal or illegal)		I'm a failure	
More accident prone than normal		I'm forgetful, I keep forgetting where I put things	

Overeating or loss of appetite	I should be able to cope
Over-reacting to situations	No one seems to understand
Poor judgement	Self-pity
Poor time management skills	What's the point?
Unable to express your feelings	Why is everyone picking on me?
Unable to relax	Why me?
Withdrawing from family/friends or becoming quiet	
Total Score:	

2. Add up the number of boxes that have a tick

3. Check your score against the analysis below

0-4 symptoms: Your score suggests that you have well developed coping strategies and techniques in place. Try to maintain this positive balance in your life. You may like to revisit this questionnaire periodically to reassure yourself that everything is still ok

5-8 symptoms: Your score suggests that you are experiencing some pressure or stress in your life. There may be certain aspects of your life where you don't cope well. Appraise your life and identify the areas that need working on. Be kind to yourself during this exercise. It's easy to beat yourself up, but this is counter-productive

9-12 symptoms: Your score suggests your coping strategies and techniques aren't working well for you. Do you actually have any coping strategies and techniques?

You need to make some changes in your life and build some coping strategies or techniques into your daily routine. Otherwise stress will become a serious threat to your health and wellbeing.

Identify the most stressful area of your life and devise an action plan to tackle this first. Don't try to tackle everything at once as this will simply add to your stress

13 or more symptoms: Stress is clearly dominant in your life right now. It's time to take action. Which issues can you address now? You can't tackle everything at once, but failure to take any action may damage your physical health and emotional wellbeing. The exercises in this book are temporary stress relievers. They probably won't make a significant difference to you, although they will help provide temporary respite

Are the problems causing your stress long-term or more than you can deal with? If so, consider getting professional help from GP or a Counsellor. Sometimes our problems are too big for us to tackle on our own

4. Now you've identified your current stress level you need to decide what you're going to do about it. Create an action plan to do address your stress level. This can include quick fixes or future strategies to ensure you have pressure not stress in your life

4.24 Identify Your Coping Strategies Exercise

At some point we all experience stress. The better we can manage it the less physical and emotional harm we will suffer. Different coping strategies work for different people.

The key to successful stress management is finding out what works for you, and then applying those strategies. You may already have tried and trusted coping strategies that you always use, but why not try something new.

Time required: 5-10 minutes

Instructions:

In the table below I have created a list of coping strategies. You may already be applying some of these. Others may be new to your or not work for you. This is OK. You can always create your own coping strategies.

Read each suggestion, and then tick the relevant box. You can return to this document as often as you need to. It's just another tool to help you conquer stress

Suggestion	I do this	Will try this	Not for me
Add a little exercise to my life (e.g. walking, cycling, yoga, Zumba, deskercise etc.)			
Avoid people who stress me out or make me feel negative			
Challenge myself to new experiences to grow			

my confidence			
Create a personal attributes list (learn to like me)			
Do something creative e.g. painting, sewing, gardening etc.			
Find a common interest group			
Find inner peace and happiness			
Get some fresh air (ideally every day for a few minutes)			
Keep in touch with friends (via text, email, telephone or face-to-face)			
Have a healthy, balanced diet			
Identify my key skills and the things I need help with			
Improve my communication skills			
I will ask family and friends for help or support when I need it			
Laugh (try to find something to laugh about every day)			
Learn to accept the things I can't control and stop stressing about it			
Learn to delegate and accept that I don't need to do everything			
Make the most of my best time of day by identifying whether I'm a lark or a night owl			
Make time for relaxation and fun in my life			
Manage my time effectively (create a to-do list or prioritise tasks)			
Meditate			
Never dwell on past mistakes			
Pamper myself			
Pet an animal			
Practice different relaxation techniques to find the right ones for me			
Practice saying no, and not feel guilty			
Read a book, magazine or kindle for a few minutes each day			
Relax more and get plenty of sleep			
See a counsellor or my GP if I need professional help			
Seek peer support when I need it			

Switch off the laptop and mobile phone outside working hours			
Take regular short breaks at work			
Use scents and aromatherapy oils to improve my mood			
Use positive affirmations to develop a positive mind-set			
Use visualisation as a problem solving tool			
Volunteer			
Write a gratitude list to remind myself of all the good things I have in my life			
Write a letter about the person/situation causing me stress, and then burn it			
Write my feelings down in a stress diary or journal			

Like stress itself, stress management is deeply personal. The more techniques you apply the less stress you will have in your life. It's important to do the things you have said you will do. Otherwise the situation won't improve. Decide when you will start this new regime and do it.

4.25 Legs And Bottom (Gluteal Muscles) Deskercises

Deskercise is a catchy name given to exercises that you can do at your desk. There are lots of different versions of deskercises available. These exercises are based on the deskercises created by author, Emily Milam. Each of these exercises is designed for the workplace, and takes just a few minutes.

We already know that physical exercise is beneficial in tackling stress. Research suggests that even deskercise can be beneficial to physical health and mental wellbeing. A short burst of deskercise will have some benefit if you're stressed as it will provide a welcome distraction for a few minutes.

Time required: 2-5 minutes per exercise

Instructions:

This set of exercises focuses on your legs and gluteal muscles. You can do just one, some, or all of these eight exercises; the choice is yours.

The Wall Sit:
Wall sits are great for building strength and endurance. Stand with your back against the wall. Now bend your knees and slide your back down the wall until the thighs are parallel to the floor. Sit and hold this position for 30-60 seconds. Repeat this at least twice.

To increase your workout try crossing the right ankle over the left knee, hold for 15 seconds, then switch! This exercise provides a great distraction as it's hard to concentrate on this and stress at the same time.

The Patient Printer:
Photocopying or standing at the printer is a great time for a quick exercise. Stand with feet shoulder-width apart. Press up onto your tippy toes, pause at the top, and then lower your feet and legs back down.

Repeat this exercise until the printing is finished. This is a great way to build a little exercise into your day. It also takes your mind off the situations/people causing you stress. The alternative is you would spend your time at the printer focusing on what is bothering you.

The Silent Seat Squeeze:
To start toning your gluteal muscles simply squeeze your buttocks. Hold for 5-10 seconds, and release. Repeat 3 times or until your gluteal muscles tire. Over time you will notice that you acquire a firmer 'butt'.

Each time you're feeling anxious about something try this exercise for a couple of minutes. This is a way of consciously deciding to do something about pressure before it takes hold. It will help you to become more aware of what stresses you.

The Seated Leg Raiser:
This is a great exercise to do while you are seated. Straighten one or both legs, raise them off the floor and hold in place up to a count of 5. Then gently lower your leg(s) back to the floor without letting your feet touch the floor. Repeat this exercise 15 times.

Each time you do this imagine yourself letting go of your stress.

If your brain is feeling clogged but you don't have time for a break try this exercise. It only takes a couple of minutes. This mini break will help clear your mind. It's an easy exercise to do each time you feel yourself starting to get tense or anxious.

The Last Man Standing:
Standing isn't exactly a traditional exercise, but research shows it has more value than just sitting. Long periods of sitting are linked to an increased risk of diabetes, obesity, and cardiovascular disease.

On the other hand, standing increases your daily calorific expenditure. Stand whenever you can.

You might like to consider standing in meetings too. This has been proven to shorten the length of meetings. This may be helpful if you're under pressure to meet tight deadlines or clear a heavy workload.

The Desk Squat:
Instead of just standing around, add a squat to your daily deskercise routine. Start by standing with your feet together (and the desk chair pushed out of the way).

Bend your knees slightly so the thighs are almost parallel to the ground, as if sitting in a chair. As you bend, raise your arms straight up or towards your computer screen. Keep your knees together and aligned. Hold for 15 seconds and then release.

Repeat this exercise at least 3 times. You might feel silly doing this exercise, but just laugh at yourself. Laughter is great for dealing with stress. It's also another way to distract yourself from what's bothering you.

The Hamstring Strengthener:
You can strengthen your hamstrings with a standing leg curl. Stand behind your chair and hold onto it for support. Before you do this exercise make sure there is nothing and no-one behind you.

Gently kick one foot back, aiming the heel of your foot for the top of your thigh. Lower the foot back down and repeat exercise with the other leg. Repeat this exercise 10 times per leg.

If it helps, with each kick imagine you're kicking one of your stressors into touch. As I've stated previously, none of these exercises are long-term stress management strategies. However, when you're feeling tense every little distraction helps.

Work Those Inner Thighs:
For this exercise you need a sealed ream of paper. Place the package between your knees and press your legs inwards. Continue squeezing, holding the paper ream in place for 30-60 seconds. As

you do this exercise imagine you're squashing the stress out of your body.

Repeat this until you feel yourself beginning to relax a little. Five minutes of distraction if often enough to help you regain a sense of perspective. With any stressful situation it's important to respond not react.

4.26 Mantra Meditation

Mantras may have no meaning at all. If they have a meaning the sound quality of the words is more important than the mantra itself.

Mantras often form part of formal meditation. However, mantras can be used while you're walking, washing the dishes, shopping, or anything else that doesn't require too much concentration.

Time required: 5-30 minutes

Instructions:

1. Choose a mantra that you're comfortable with. Here are some mantra examples to get you started.

Modern Mantras:

Love is the only miracle there is (Osho)

Be the change you wish to see in the world (Gandhi)

Every day in every way I'm getting better and better (Laura Silva)

I change my thoughts; I change my world (Norman Vincent Peale)

Move over stress, I haven't got time for this (Liz Tucker)

Mantras from the Ancients:

Aum (pronounced Om) - is an ancient mantra but commonly used today. You really can't mess this one up too badly. The "Om" is a sacred sound in Hinduism and is said to mean, 'It Is, Will Be or To Become'

Om Mani Padme Hum – this one's a bit of a mouthful. It's from Tibet and it means, roughly, "Hail the Jewel in the Lotus." The jewel in this case is the Buddha of Compassion

Namo Amita Bha – Homage to the Buddha of boundless light

I am that I am – This is one of the Hebrew Torah's most famous lines. It was God's answer to Moses when Moses asked for his name

Ham-Sah – The Hindu variant, meaning 'I am that'

I love you, I'm sorry, Please forgive me, Thank you (Hawaiian) Mantra

2. Start by breathing deeply and exhaling slowly. Keep repeating this deep breathing until you feel relaxed

3. As you get into the rhythm of your breathing start repeating your mantra silently, or out loud if you prefer

4. Immerse yourself in the rhythm of your mantra. If you're doing this correctly you will feel the rhythm running through your body

5. If you find yourself losing focus, say the syllables more precisely

6. Keep repeating your deep breathing and saying your mantra for as long as you wish

7. When you're ready, sit quietly for 1 minute and then return to your normal activities

Like deep breathing, mantas are great for a short stress break. If you focus on the mantra and nothing else, your stressful situation doesn't get chance to run riot in your mind.

4.27 Measure Your Current Stress Level Exercise

Recognising stress symptoms and how often they occur is a good way to start dealing with your stress. Knowing your current stress level is very helpful. This will tell you whether you just need to make small lifestyle changes or need help from a medical professional.

This exercise is based on what has happened in the previous 4-6 weeks. Read each of the stress symptoms in the table below. Identify how often you have experienced each of them in the last few weeks.

Time required: 20 minutes

Instructions:

1. Read each stress symptom in the table below and give it a score of 0 - 4

Stress symptom scale:

0 = Never

1 = Sometimes

2 = Often

3 = Frequently

Symptom	Score
Accident prone	
Aching neck or shoulders	
Anger/bad tempered	
Change of sex drive	
Cold hands or feet	
Colds or flu	
Constantly unwell (this can be viruses, stomach upsets or anything else that makes you feel unwell)	
Diarrhoea or constipation	
Difficulty concentrating	
Dry mouth or throat	
Everything feels like hard work	
Excessive or significantly increased smoking	
Excessive spending	
Fatigue or tiredness	
Feelings of helplessness or hopelessness	
Feelings of sadness	
Feeling restless	
Feeling tired	
Feeling upset/crying	
Forgetfulness	
Frequent absences from work	
Gritted teeth or clenched jaw	
Headaches or migraines	
Heartburn or indigestion	
Hives or skin rash	
Impatience	
Increased alcohol intake	
Increased perspiration	
Irritability	
Joint pain	
Lack of energy	
Lower or upper back pain	
Moody	
Nail biting	
Nausea	
Nervousness or anxiety	
Not drinking enough water	
Not eating or not eating regularly	

Not enjoying time with family and friends	
Overeating	
Poor diet (junk food)	
Pounding heart or irregular heartbeat	
Racing or intrusive thoughts (can't still your mind)	
Rapid breathing	
Rapid pulse	
Significant increase in medication or drug use	
Sleeping difficulties (nightmares, can't sleep)	
Tightness in your chest	
Twitches or nervous tic	
Unkind to others	
Worrying a lot/fretful	
Your total stress-symptom score	

2. Add up each of your scores to give you a total score. Look at the stress rating table below to identify your current stress level

Your Score	Your Comparative Rating
0–19	Lower than average
20–39	Average
40–49	Moderately higher than average
50 and above	Much higher than average

3. Below you will see the analysis relating to your stress rating:

Lower than average: If your score is lower than average, enjoy this time. Your score suggests that you have well developed coping strategies and techniques in place. Give yourself a pat on the back.

Average: Your score suggests that you manage some of your stressors well. There may be certain aspects of your life where you don't cope well. Look at your life and identify the areas that need working on. Some quick fixes may be all you need.

Moderately higher than average: This score suggests your coping strategies and techniques aren't working for you, or work sporadically. Do you actually have any coping strategies and techniques, or are you allowing stress to happen to you? Maybe you are too busy fighting the fire to actually tackle the underlying issues.

You need to take stock. Build some coping strategies/techniques into your daily life before stress becomes a serious threat to your health and wellbeing.

Much higher than average: Whoa, it's time to take action. You clearly have some issues that need addressing now. Failure to take action is likely to damage your physical health and emotional wellbeing.

In the first instance try the Problem Solving Exercise, Problem Solving Visualisation, the Centring Technique Exercise or a meditation. None of these will fix all your problems, but they will give you a little temporary respite from your stressors. Use the stress break to think about your long-term stress relief strategy.

Are the problems causing this level of stress long-term or more than you can deal with? If so, consider seeing your GP or a Counsellor. Prolonged stress is not good for your physical, mental or emotional health.

Note: If your score is 50 or above consult your GP. This is just a precaution in case there are any other factors besides stress that are involved.

4. Now you know what your current stress level is. So, what you're going to do about it? Consider any quick fixes you could apply to your life right now. Anything that will provide you with some temporary stress relief is a good starting point.

Consider learning to delegate tasks at home or at work. Going for a walk 2-3 times a week, practicing deep breathing or stretching exercises every day may help reduce stress.

Consider what you are willing to do to reduce your stress level. Don't make promises you have no intention of keeping as this will simply add to your stress level. Doing nothing is not an option if you're serious about tackling your stress level.

4.28 Mindfulness Relaxation Technique

Focusing on the past, blaming and judging yourself, or worrying about the future can lead to stress or increase your stress level. By staying calm and focused in the present moment, you can bring your nervous system back into balance.

Mindfulness can be applied to activities such as walking, exercising, eating, or meditation. "My advice to anyone would be to spend at least five minutes every day practising mindfulness" says Linda Blair, Clinical Psychologist.

Time required: 5-30 minutes

Instructions:

1. Choose a quiet place in your home, office, garden, or somewhere outdoors where you can relax without distractions or interruptions

2. Get comfortable, but don't lie down as this may lead to you falling asleep. Sit up with your spine straight, either in a chair or on the floor. Alternatively, you can sit in the lotus position

3. Breathe in deeply through your nose. Hold your breath for a count of 3-5 and then exhale very slowly through your mouth

4. Repeat this breathing exercise for a couple of minutes until you feel yourself starting to relax

5. Now select a point to focus on. This point can be internal or external. An internal point can be a feeling or imaginary scene. An external point could be a picture, flame, a word or phrase (that you repeat throughout the exercise)

6. Keep breathing deeply. As you breathe focus on your chosen object. For example, if you have chosen a candle flame - keep your mind focused on the flickering flame. In your mind see this and nothing else

7. Repeat this breathing and mindfulness exercise until you feel ready to resume your normal activities. The longer you spend on this exercise the greater benefit you will experience

8. When you have finished the exercise sit quietly for a minute. Notice how you feel now. Do you feel calmer? Is your mind less frantic? Do you feel relaxed?

9. When you feel ready, resume your normal activities

Note: It's important to adopt an observant, noncritical attitude. Don't worry about any distracting thoughts that go through your mind, and don't worry about how well you're doing.

If thoughts pop into your head during your relaxation session, don't fight them. Instead, acknowledge them, allow the thought to go and then gently turn your attention back to your point of focus.

4.29 Mini Self Massage

You may not have the time or money for a professional massage so why not give yourself a mini-massage. This massage is based on Darrin Zeer's Lover's Massage and Office Yoga Technique. Enjoy!

Time required: 5-10 minutes

Instructions:
1. Place your hands on your shoulders and neck. If you're very tense this may not be comfortable to do. If you practice this regularly the tension will lessen

2. Squeeze your shoulders and neck with your palms, thumbs and fingers. Repeat this 5 times

3. If you can't do both shoulders at once, tackle one side and then the other

4. Vigorously rub each shoulder for 1 minute. Rub one shoulder at a time

5. Wrap one hand around the top of your other arm. Gently squeeze the muscles with your thumb and fingers

6. Move your thumb and fingers down the length of your arm; squeezing gently as you go. This may be a little uncomfortable initially. As you relax it will feel more comfortable

7. Repeat this step 3 times

8. Now switch arms and repeat steps 5, 6 and 7

9. Vigorously rub each arm in turn for 1 minute

10. Shake your arms and hands. Now you're ready to return to your normal activities

4.30 My Life, My Stress Exercise

This exercise is designed to show you how well, or not, you are able to deal with a particular situation. Just pick one stressor for this exercise. You can always repeat the exercise for other stressors in your life.

Time required: 10–15 minutes

Instructions:

1. Think of a single problem that is causing you stress currently. Your stressor could be an issue to do with work, your spouse, family, financial or personal matters, or anything else. Visualise the problem

in as much detail as possible as this will help you to answer the questions below

2. Read each of the helpful behaviour statements in the table below. For each statement, tick the most relevant box. For example, I sit and think about issues to help me put things into perspective. Your answer may be 'periodically'

Helpful Behaviour	Never	Rarely	Periodically	Regularly	Frequently
I sit and think about issues to help me put things into perspective					
I learn something from every stressful situation					
I'm comfortable talking to someone who can do something about the problem/issue					
I feel able to cry in front of family or close friends					
I'm happy to talk about my feelings with people I trust					
Although I get angry with people or situations that cause me stress, I'm able to release these thoughts afterwards					
I'm able to see when I'm over dramatizing a situation					
I am able to accept that some things are beyond my control					
Somewhat Helpful Behaviour					
I share my problems/issues with various people whether they can help me or not					
I go over problems in my mind again and again to help me to understand, but I know when to stop					

	Never	Rarely	Periodically	Regularly	Frequently
I always try to get empathy or understanding from someone who isn't directly involved					

3. Look at your responses to the helpful and somewhat helpful behaviours. Give yourself a pat on the back for the ticks in the 'regularly or frequently' columns

4. Now look at the ticks in the 'never, rarely or periodically' columns. What are you going to do to about this? These are clearly problem areas for you. It's important to take action as the problem won't simply go away

5. Now read each of the unhelpful behaviour statements below. For each statement, tick the most relevant box. The responses you tick today may be different in six months' time if you repeat this exercise. Your answers are based on how you feel right now

Unhelpful Behaviour	Never	Rarely	Periodically	Regularly	Frequently
I try to block problems out of my mind as I don't want to face up to them					
When I'm stressed I often go quiet and withdrawn					
I try to pretend nothing has happened and continue as normal. Other people rarely know when I'm feeling under pressure or stressed					
I prefer to be left alone when I'm under pressure or stressed					
I feel very uncomfortable discussing my feelings and so prefer to keep things to myself					
When I'm suffering from stress I worry a lot, and sometimes exaggerate the problem in my own mind					
I often have sleeping problems when I'm stressed					

My eating habits change when I'm stressed (I either eat too much or stop eating properly)					
I keep revisiting the past, wishing I could change what has happened					
I imagine how things might have turned out if I had done things differently					
I don't cry or show emotion in front of other people					
I talk to anyone and everyone about my stressors, even if I run the risk of repeating myself to the same people					

6. Look at your responses to the unhelpful behaviours. Give yourself a pat on the back for the statements where you have ticked 'never, rarely or periodically'

7. Now look at the 'regularly or frequently' columns. Decide what you're going to do about this. These behaviours are clearly challenging you, and are probably exacerbating your stress level. It's important to tackle this. Failure to act will increase your stress level

4.31 Neck Stretch Exercise

This quick exercise can be done anywhere (including your desk) and at any time. All you need is a chair. If you're very tense you may find this exercise quite painful to start with.

As you become more relaxed the exercise will feel more comfortable. This will be a clear indicator that you are successfully reducing your tension level.

Try to build this exercise into your daily routine. Your neck will be grateful.

Time required: 5-10 minutes

Instructions:

1. This exercise works best is you keep your shoulder down as you lean away from it. Sit comfortably and put your hands on your thighs

2. Extend your upper body and drop your chin onto your chest. Return your head back to the starting position. Now drop your shoulders

3. Tilt your head towards your left shoulder. Hold your head in this position for a count of 3-5. Return to your starting position. Repeat this 3 times

4. Tilt your head towards your right shoulder. Hold your head in this position for a count of 3-5. Return to your starting position. Repeat this 3 times

5. Tilt your head towards your left shoulder. Place your right hand on the right side of your head, and press your head down towards your shoulder. This will increase the stretch. Hold this position for as long as you feel comfortable. Return to your starting position

6. Tilt your head towards your right shoulder. Place your left hand on the left side of your head, and press your head down towards your shoulder. Hold this position for as long as you feel comfortable. Return to your starting position

7. Turn your head towards your left side. Tilt your head towards your chest. Hold your head in this position for a count of 3-5. Return to your starting position

8. Turn your head towards your right side. Tilt your head towards your chest. Hold your head in this position for a count of 3-5. Return to your starting position

9. Finally, clasp your hands behind your head and push your head backwards while resisting with your hands. Hold this position for a count of 3-5

4.32 Powernap Exercise

Do you find yourself nodding off during the afternoon slump? Perhaps you sometimes feel drowsy when driving, or during a night shift. A powernap might be the answer.

Scientists advise that power napping can make you more alert and productive, but only if you do it correctly.

Time required: 15-30 minutes

Instructions:

1. Approximately 20 minutes before your powernap have a cup of coffee (or another source of caffeine). I know this sounds counter intuitive, but it won't kick-in immediately. This will lessen how sleepy you feel after your powernap

2. Find a good place for your powernap. Turn off your mobile phone and any other distractions

3. Set the alarm to go off in 15-30 minutes time (depending how long you want to sleep)

4. Settle down and tell your mind it's going to sleep. If you have difficulty sleeping initially, use the time to close your eyes and relax or meditate. Not everyone can slip into power napping at first

You can buy CDs or soundtracks that are designed to induce a sleep state

5. By the time your alarm goes off the caffeine should have been absorbed. Open your eyes and resume your activities immediately. If you sleep longer than 30 minutes you may feel groggy when you wake up

4.33 Problem Solving Exercise

Gaining control over even a small part of your life is very empowering. The feeling of having a sense of control helps reduce stress.

The best way to solve problems is to tackle them one at a time. Never try to tackle all your problems or issues in one go. A long list of problems and stressors will make you feel worse rather than better.

For this exercise choose a single situation that is causing you stress right now. All you need for this exercise is a pen and a piece of paper.

Time required: up to 30 minutes

Instructions:

1. Give your problem/stressor a name e.g. workplace bully, financial problems, relationship issues etc

2. Write down exactly what the problem is. Write this in as much detail as possible. I know this may be painful but it's all part of the releasing process

3. List every possible solution you can think of. It doesn't matter whether you like the potential solution or not. The point of this exercise is to view your stressor as broadly as possible

4. Next, objectively weigh up the pros and cons of each solution. If it helps, imagine this is someone else's problem and you're trying to help them

5. Choose the option that suits your needs best. This might not be your preferred option, but it is the option that is the most suitable solution. Your ability to do this will demonstrate your willingness to resolve the situation. Often we hang onto problems, for whatever reasons

6. Create an action plan. This plan is all the steps you need to go through to make this solution work for you. Try to make these small, easily achievable goals. Lots of small goals are better than one big one

7. Implement your plan

8. Each time you achieve one of your mini goals reward yourself in some way. This could be 10 minutes reading a book, a small bar of chocolate or a small gift etc. It really doesn't matter what your reward is. The important thing is to give yourself a pat on the back for taking another step closer to solving the problem

You can apply this process to each stressor or major issue in your life. Empowerment is great for helping reduce stress as it gives you a sense of control.

4.34 Problem Solving Visualisation Exercise

Whether we're aware of it or not we often use visualisation to solve problems. Sometimes we create an image of the situation that is bothering us in order to make sense of it.

Do you ever find yourself overanalysing your problems? This is a very common trait but it isn't helpful. There's a fine line between analysing a problem to find and solution and overanalysing it and making matters worse.

If you're new to the problem solving visualisation technique it may feel awkward initially. Many people new to this technique report finding it hard to concentrate as their mind keeps wandering. This is normal so don't beat yourself up!

When your mind wanders simply acknowledge the thought. Then bring your thoughts back to the problem you want to focus on. Visualisation gets easier and more effective the more you do it.

Visualisation works best if you can do it in a fairly quiet place, without distractions. I have created this exercise based on sitting somewhere quiet.

You may choose to do this exercise sitting in a chair, standing, while out walking or anywhere else you feel comfortable. Do what you feel most comfortable with. Personally, I go for a walk when I want to do this exercise.

Tackle your problems just one at a time. Never be tempted to deal with all your problems in a single visualisation exercise as it doesn't work.

Time required: 10-30 minutes

Instructions:

1. Find somewhere quiet to do this exercise. Sit down in a chair, with your back straight. Make sure your feet are on the floor and your hands are relaxed in your lap. If you're standing or walking to do this exercise make sure your back is straight and your head held high

2. Breathe in deeply, through your nose. Hold your breath up to a count of 3-5. Slowly exhale through your mouth

3. Repeat this deep breathing for a couple of minutes or until you start to feel relaxed

4. Now you're ready to begin your problem solving visualisation. Visualise a single personal or work situation that is causing you some anxiety, pressure or stress

5. Visualise the situation in as much detail as possible. Imagine you're telling someone a story. Identify all the aspects of the situation that are worrying you. For example, what the problem is, who is involved, how it makes you feel, how much control you have over the situation etc.

The more detail you can include in your visualisation the better. This will help you to clear the clutter from your mind

6. Now imagine this is someone else's problem and they have come to you for advice. If this was someone else's problem what would your advice to them be?

Would you suggest more than one way to resolve the problem? Would you simply tell them how to deal with it, by not giving them options? Would you tell them it's beyond their control, and so they must learn to accept the situation?

7. Next, visualise your action plan in as much detail as possible. Think about - who, how, when etc. The clearer the picture in your mind the better the results will be

8. Now visualise yourself successfully handling the situation. See yourself tackling each part of the problem in turn. As you tackle each issue feel yourself getting stronger and the pressure reducing

9. Keep going until you've mentally resolved the problem or at least got in under control. Now you've got your problem into perspective it's important to give yourself a verbal pat on the back. Say "well done, keep up the good work"

10. Write a brief summary of the problem and how you plan to tackle it. You don't need to spend any more time worrying about it as you now have a plan. Your energy should be directed towards your plan

Note: If you have worked through this exercise systematically you should feel more positive. You should be able to return to your normal activities with a clear idea of how you're going to approach the problem.

4.35 Progressive Muscle Relaxation Exercise

Do not attempt this exercise if you suffer from muscle spasms or back problems. These health problems may be aggravated by tensing your muscles.

Progressive muscle relaxation involves systematically tensing and relaxing different muscle groups in your body. The end result is a much less tense body.

You may not be able to do this exercise for all the muscle groups initially. This is fine, do what you can. With practice you will be able to do each muscle group.

Time required: 30-45 minutes

Instructions:

1. Loosen your clothing, take off your shoes, and sit comfortably. Get into a position where your spine is fairly straight and your feet are on the floor

2. Breathe in deeply through your nose. Hold your breath for a count of 3-5. Then exhale very slowly through your mouth

3. Repeat this breathing exercise for a couple of minutes until you feel yourself starting to relax

4. When you're relaxed and ready to start, shift your attention to your right foot. Take a moment to focus on the way it feels

5. Now, slowly tense the muscles in your right foot. Squeeze them as tightly as you can. Hold for a count of 5-10 and then relax your right foot. Stop if it feels painful. Notice the tension flowing away and the way your foot feels as it becomes limp and loose

Note: If you're left-handed you may prefer to begin with your left foot instead

6. Stay in this relaxed state for a moment, breathing deeply and slowly

7. When you're ready, shift your attention to your left foot. Repeat steps 5 and 6 on your left foot

8. Move slowly up through your body, contracting and relaxing each muscle group as you go. Here is the progressive muscle relaxation sequence:

Right foot

Left foot

Right calf
Left calf
Right thigh
Left thigh
Hips and buttocks
Stomach
Chest
Back (lower and upper back)
Right arm and hand
Left arm and hand
Neck and shoulders
Face and head

9. When you have completed the exercise site quietly for 1 minute. Use this time to observe how you feel

10. When you're ready resume your activities

Note: Try not to tense muscles other than those you are working on. If you find yourself getting distracted, acknowledge the thought, allow it to drift away and then return to the exercise.

4.36 Putting Yourself To Sleep Exercise

Sleep is often hard to achieve when you're feeling stressed. Once you have started to reduce your daily stress levels, you will find that sleep comes more easily. This is another good reason to get your stress under control.

Stress is very tiring. If you are very stressed you may wake up feeling as tired as you were when you went to bed. This just makes you feel worse. You may find that with less stress you need less sleep.

Meditation techniques can help to get you into a sleep state. You may find soothing music playing quietly helps with this exercise.

Time required: As long as it takes

Instructions:

1. Get into bed and get settled. Lie comfortably with your arms at your sides and your legs uncrossed. Just breathe normally

2. When you're ready, start. Say "toes go to sleep". As you say this, feel your toes relaxing

3. Say "feet go to sleep". As you say this, feel your feet relaxing

4. Work your way up through your body. Tell each part of your body in turn to go to sleep

5. If you find a part of your body that is holding onto tension, focus on it a little longer. Try deep breathing and seeing each deep breath soothing the tension out of this part of your body

6. You may fall asleep before you finish your entire body. This is good; it just means you have relaxed enough to sleep

7. As you start to drift into sleep you may feel yourself sinking into the bed. It might feel like a blanket gently pressing down on you. Don't try to break out of this, just drift into sleep

4.37 Put Your Feet Up Exercise

This exercise is a classic yoga pose. It soothes the nervous system and promotes deep relaxation of the mind and body. You don't need any special equipment for this exercise; just a wall.

Time required: 5 minutes

Instructions:

1. Lie on your back, on the floor. Rest your feet on the wall (as you probably did when you were a child)

2. Gently shuffle your bottom forward to the base of the wall. Your legs (not your feet) should now be resting up the wall

3. Make sure you feel comfortable in this position

4. Relax your arms by your side. Now close your eyes and breathe deeply and slowly

5. Remain in this position for 5 minutes; continuing to breathe deeply and slowly. Allow any thoughts you have to just come and go. Don't hold onto your thoughts or analyse them

6. When you're ready, slowly get up and continue with your day. Notice how much better you feel after this quick stress busting break

4.38 Quick Dealing With Nerves Exercise

This is a short deep breathing exercise that you might like to try when you are feeling anxious or nervous. It works on connecting your breathing with your solar plexus. This exercise can be helpful when you're going to a job interview.

This exercise only takes a couple of minutes, and can be done anywhere.

Time required: 2 minutes - or as long as necessary

Instructions:

1. Find your solar plexus. This is situated two inches below your breastbone. It is in the centre of your body, behind your stomach

2. Place the palms of your hands across your stomach. Your thumbs should be pointing upwards. Your middle fingers should be touching, and should be over your solar plexus

3. Breathe in through your nose. Breathe as deeply as you possibly can. This breath should expand your lungs and diaphragm. If your shoulders move you're not breathing deeply enough

4. Slowly exhale through your mouth. Force as much air out as you can

5. Keep your hands in place and repeat this exercise at least 5 times. You may prefer to keep doing this until you start to relax

6. Notice how much calmer your feel. Now you're ready to resume your activities

4.39 Reclaiming Yourself Meditation

This is a good weekend or holiday exercise. Far too often we focus our energy on the wellbeing of others and neglect our own needs. It's important to start the weekend or holiday by paying attention to your needs.

This visualisation exercise is about reclaiming all the energy you have expended on others over the week. This is also a useful exercise if you have had a very difficult or tiring day.

Time required: 5-15 minutes

Instructions:

1. Find somewhere comfortable to sit. Try to choose somewhere you won't be disturbed for a few minutes

2. Close your eyes and breathe in deeply. Hold your breath for a count of 3-5. Slowly breathe out. Repeat this 2 or 3 times

3. Think about the people or projects that have claimed your time and energy this week. Visualise a cord of energy running from your body to each person or project. You may end up with lots of cords of energy. This is fine; it's just a reminder of how thinly you have spread yourself

4. Keep breathing deeply. As you do this, systematically pull all this energy back into your body. Keep doing this until all the cords have been broken. If you find it hard to do this, imagine using a fishing rod. As you turn the reel on your fishing rod, you pull all this energy back into you

5. Once all your cords are broken rest for a moment. See yourself filled with beautiful energy. Slowly open your eyes

6. Sit quietly for 1 minute. Don't say anything during this minute. When you feel ready, resume your normal activities. Before you do so, notice how much lighter you feel

4.40 Reflective Meditation

Reflective meditation is a systematic investigation of a single word. Imagine your chosen word is 'Joy'. As part of your meditation you will start to think about all the things that come to mind when you hear the word joy. For example

1. Occasions when you have experienced joy

2. What joy means to you. What are the words that you conjure up when you think about joy?

3. Any negative or irritating thoughts you have a about joy or joyous people

4. Keep going until you have thought of everything you possibly can about joy

Now you've got the idea have a go at this meditation.

Time required: 10-15 minutes

Instructions:

1. Select one of the following words (or a word of your choosing if you don't like any of these). These words have been specifically chosen as 'potential seed ideas' that unfold cosmic energy within you.

CALM - CHEERFULNESS - CLARITY - COMPASSION - COOPERATION - COURAGE - CREATIVITY - ENERGY - FREEDOM - GENEROSITY - GRATITUDE - HARMONY - HONESTY - HUMOUR - INCLUSIVENESS - INTEGRITY - INTUITION - JOY - LOVE - LOYALTY - MEDITATION - OPENNESS - PEACE - PLAYFULNESS - POWER - REFLECTION - RISK - SELF-WILL - SIMPLICITY - STEADFASTNESS - STRENGTH - TENACITY - TRUTHFULNESS - UNDERSTANDING - VITALITY - WISDOM - WONDER

2. Reflect on the word you have chosen. Roll it around in your head. Allow your thoughts about this chosen word to come and go. Look at the example above if you need a little help

3. When you feel you have explored this word thoroughly finish your meditation

4. Let the word go and go back to your activities. Alternatively, you might like to spend a few minutes making notes of your observations

5. Once you have mastered the art of focusing on a single word, you might like to choose phrases to meditate on. Try to choose a phrase that requires deep thought. For example 'Gratefulness is heaven itself' - William Blake

Note: It is normal to get bored with your word, or feel you have exhausted it quite quickly. Do not be tempted to stop. This is the very point at which you should stick with the exercise as it will now test you.

If you can go through and beyond this point your mind will shift into a different level. You will experience a more meaningful and lucid quality of thought. This is known as reaching a spiritual level.

4.41 Relaxation Exercise For Your Eyes

We often don't think about needing a relaxation exercise for our eyes. Working at a computer screen, reading for long periods or working in very bright or dim lighting can strain your eyes.

Generally the symptoms are sore eyes, headaches, fatigue or just feeling irritable. It's time for a quick break.

You can do this short exercise wherever you are, and can spend just 2-3 minutes or 30 minutes; the choice is yours.

Time required: 2-30 minutes

Instructions:

1. Sit down in a chair and put down anything you have in your hands. Get into a comfortable position where your spine is fairly straight and your feet are on the floor

2. With your eyes open, sit with your head squarely on your shoulders (not tilted to one side or backwards or forwards). Open your eyes as wide as you can and look straight ahead

3. Without moving your head raise your eyes towards the ceiling. Hold this position and count to 5. Return your eyes to your starting position (looking straight ahead)

4. Continue to keep your head still. Now, roll your eyes to the right and focus on something e.g. the wall, a picture, ornament etc. Slowly count to 5. Return your eyes to your starting position

5. Next, roll your eyes to the left and focus on something e.g. the wall, a picture, ornament etc. Slowly count to 5. Return your eyes to your starting position

6. Roll your eyes downwards. Hold this position and count to 5. Return your eyes to your starting position

7. Roll your eyes upwards again. Count to 5 while your eyes are in this position. Return to your starting position

8. Keep repeating this exercise until your eyes feel less sore or you're ready to resume what you were doing

9. Finally, close your eyes. Let your head and shoulders relax. Rest in this position 1 minute

10. Resume your activities. Notice how much better your eyes feel

4.42 Relaxation Sequence Exercise

This is a good follow-on exercise for anyone who has already mastered the art of deep breathing. Everyone can benefit from this exercise, in varying degrees as it works on systematically relaxing each part of your body. This exercise is very similar to the progressive muscle relaxation exercise.

All you need is a chair for this exercise. It is possible to do this exercise lying down if you prefer. This exercise is wonderful whenever you need to relax. It doesn't take a lot of time, but you will feel the benefits of it immediately.

You can skip through this exercise in less than 10 minutes, but you will find it more beneficial if you work through it slowly. Just relax and enjoy it.

Time required: 10-20 minutes

Instructions:

1. Sit down in a chair. Put down anything you have in your hands and remove your shoes. Get into a comfortable position where your spine is fairly straight. The first part of this exercise is done with your eyes open

2. Start with your feet. Curl your toes and press your feet down into the floor. Stop if you find this painful. Now slowly relax your toes. Repeat this 2 or 3 times

3. Press your heels down into the floor and bend your feet upwards. Now slowly relax your feet. Repeat this 2 or 3 times

4. Tense your calf muscles and then slowly relax them. Repeat this 2 or 3 times. If you can't master this step just carry on to the next one

5. Tense your thigh muscles, straightening your knees and making your legs stiff. Now slowly relax your thigh muscles. Repeat this 2 or 3 times

6. Clench your buttocks so they feel tense and then slowly relax them. Repeat this 2 or 3 times

7. Tense your stomach (as if you're about to receive a punch). Hold your muscles tense to a count of 5. Slowly relax your stomach muscles. Repeat this 2 or 3 times

8. Bend your elbows and tense your arm muscles. Hold your arms in this position to a count of 5. Now slowly relax your arm muscles and straighten your elbows. Repeat this 2 or 3 times

9. Hunch your shoulders and push your chest out. If you are lying down hunch your shoulders and push your head back into a cushion or pillow. Slowly relax. Repeat this 2 or 3 times

10. Tip your head back (so your chin is jutting out and the front of your neck feels taut). Gently tilt your head and neck to the left and then to the right. Slowly relax your head and neck muscles. This may be uncomfortable to start with. Repeat this at least 2 or 3 times.

You may like to do this step more times if your neck and shoulders muscles are particularly tense

11. Clench your jaw shut tightly, frown and screw up your eyes. Now gently relax your face muscles. Repeat this 2 or 3 times

12. Close your eyes, breathe in deeply and then slowly exhale. Repeat this 2 or 3 times

13. Continue with your deep breathing. Now imagine a beautiful white rose on a black background. See the rose very clearly. Is it fully open, or tightly in bud? Notice how perfect the petals are. Focus on this rose for approximately 1 minute

14. Continue to keep your eyes closed. Choose another image that you find peaceful. For example, waves lapping against the shoreline, hot air balloon, another flower, water fountain, a colour etc

15. Tell yourself that when you open your eyes you will feel perfectly relaxed and alert

16. When you're ready slowly open your eyes. Notice how relaxed you feel. Sit quietly for 1 minute before resuming your activities

17. Whenever you start to feel tense take your mind back to your anchor image. This can be the rose or your other image. Allow this to soothe you. This anchor image is a useful thought to use every time you notice yourself become anxious or tense

4.43 Ritual Departure Exercise

Are you one of those people who mentally or physically take work home with you? Creating a little ritual for leaving work makes it easier to leave work issues at work.

It's important for your physical, emotional and mental wellbeing to be able to separate work from other parts of your life. If you don't have a mental break from work you won't be fresh when you go to work the next day.

Time required: 5-10 minutes

Instructions:

1. Breathe in deeply. Hold your breath to a count of 3-5 and then exhale slowly. Repeat this twice more

2. Now start to tidy up your desk or work area. As you do this, continue to breathe deeply

3. Put things away e.g. pens, folders, equipment etc. It's important to do this even if you normally leave things where they are. This ritual is all part of mentally switching off from work

4. As you put things away, emotionally detach yourself as if you no longer need this item. This is called letting go of the energy connection. This may feel strange at first but stick with it. This gets easier with regular practice

5. As you put things away see the energy reeling back into your hands

6. Now pack your bag, briefcase etc and put on your coat. As you put your coat on, imagine work falling off your shoulders and dropping onto the floor. Imagine your work has now formed a puddle in the middle of the floor

7. Take a final deep breath. Now step over your 'work puddle' and see yourself leaving this pile of work behind. Know it will still be here waiting for you tomorrow

8. Walk out the door. As you go through the doorway imagine a blast of light showering down onto you. This light is giving you some new energy for the rest of the day/evening ahead

9. Keep walking and don't think about work, or what you've left behind. Focus on the rest of your day/evening instead

Note: If you do this ritual daily, you will find it becomes natural very quickly. Your productivity at work will also increase. It's essential for effective stress management to be able to let go for a while.

4.44 Roll Your Shoulders Exercise

Your shoulders are one of the most flexible joints in your body, when they are functioning smoothly. When you're stressed your shoulders can feel like boulders.

To keep your shoulders flexible do this shoulder roll at least three times a day. This exercise can be done one shoulder at a time or both shoulders together, and it only takes a couple of minutes.

Time required: 2 minutes

Instructions:

1. Stand or sit tall in your chair
2. Lift your shoulders as high as you can
3. Bring your shoulders forward
4. Push your shoulders down
5. Next, pull your shoulders back and then return to the starting position
6. Repeat this exercise at least 10 times or until your shoulders feel less tense

4.45 Secret Garden Guided Meditation

This is designed to be a guided meditation. Ideally you want to find someone with a soothing voice to lead you through this guided meditation. Alternatively, read the instructions and imagine the secret garden sequence.

This meditation takes approximately 20-30 minutes. Don't worry the time will pass quickly.

Time required: Approximately 20-30 minutes

Instructions:

1. Sit comfortably in your seat and allow your shoulders to drop
2. Close your eyes. You're always in control so you can return to your awakened state at any time by simply opening your eyes
3. Now get rid of any preconceived ideas you have about meditation and just approach this with an open mind. The worst thing that will happen is you'll think it's boring or not for me. Hopefully you will enjoy the experience and feel relaxed at the end of it
4. Take a deep breath. Try to breathe right down to your stomach. You may find it hard to breathe this deeply to start with but just breathe as deeply as you can
5. Now exhale (breathe out) very slowly
6. Repeat this deep breathing 5 times

7. Breathe in deeply and exhale once more. As you breathe out this time feel your arms, legs and body become relaxed. Know that you are perfectly safe and in control

8. Continue to breathe in deeply and exhale slowly

9. Each time you exhale imagine releasing one of your worries. If you can't let go of a particular thought make a mental note to deal with it later

10. Continue breathing in and out, releasing all your worries and anxieties

11. Notice the sense of peace, tranquillity and contentment you're feeling right now. All your worries are disappearing for a little while, as this is your relaxation time

12. Imagine it's a warm summer's day and you're standing in a beautiful garden by a water fountain

13. The fountain is carved from stone. See yourself watching the crystal clear water trickling over the fountain. Notice how soothing it is as it washes away your cares

14. As you look around you notice your secret garden is surrounded by a lovely old stone wall. You know you are safe and can be peaceful in this secret space of yours. This wall is here to protect you

15. This is your private place. You can come here anytime you like. It's where you can escape the demands of your daily life

16. This is your time now and here in your secret garden no one expects anything of you. You can simply enjoy a few minutes of 'me-time' to recharge your batteries

17. On the other side of the lawn you notice two large beautiful oak trees. They have been here for hundreds of years, and store many secrets. In the shade between these trees is a hammock - just waiting for you

18. Notice the warm sunshine filling your body with soothing heat. It's not too hot - just the right temperature

19. Slowly make your way across the lawn to your hammock. As you walk notice how lovely the lawn looks. You realise that someone has given a lot of time and love to make this lawn look beautiful for you

20. Climb into your hammock and make yourself comfortable

21. Look around you and enjoy this place of peace and beauty. Notice the beautiful flowers and shrubs. All of this belongs to you. No one can share this with you or take it from you

22. Notice how relaxed your body feels. You probably can't remember the last time you felt this relaxed and at peace with the world. Just enjoy it - this is your time

23. Use your senses to take it all in. Notice the weather, the environment, wildlife, plants and trees. Can you hear the birds singing? Can you smell the scent from any of the flowers? Notice everything you can about your environment, and know it's all here for you

24. Take as long as you like to explore this special place. It's yours to enjoy, and you have all the time in the world

25. Notice how you feel right now. The peace and tranquillity is just what you needed today. Your body needed this time to relax and be peaceful

26. Take a few minutes to enjoy the beauty of your surroundings. Your day-to-day life seems so far away. None of it matters right now - you can deal with it later. I'm going to stop talking for a minute or two. Just take this time focus on the peace and beauty of where you are. Be silent for a couple of minutes

27. From this safe place look at one of the issues that have been troubling you. What's been causing you stress or anxiety? Is it work related, financial, are you struggling to communicate with your children, are you having relationship problems? Choose just one thing that's bothering you

28. If nothing's bothering you right now, think about something good in your life that you don't normally have time to appreciate. Perhaps you've had a wonderful holiday or just got married. Take time to reflect on this

29. Going back to your problem, give this issue or event a name. For example, nightmare time at work, or challenging teenagers etc

30. Repeat this name in your mind

31. Now look at the issue or event. Observe your thoughts and feelings from this safe place. Don't try to control your thoughts just notice what you see and feel. Allow your thoughts to come and go as you breathe. Is this issue going to matter in 3 months' time? Will it matter one year from now? Is it really important enough to cause you so much anxiety?

32. This session will be ending shortly so prepare to leave this issue or event for now. Have you come to any conclusions? It doesn't matter if you haven't as this space has given you chance to look at the issue more objectively. The answer will come to you in due course

33. Say goodbye to the topic you've been observing. Say goodbye "nightmare time at work, challenging teenagers" or whatever you called your issue/event

34. Now look at the beautiful oak trees supporting your hammock. Wonder about the many secrets they hold and their history. Look at how strong they are. You are like an oak tree - you're strong and can deal with all your issues

35. Look at the sky above you and see the lovely fluffy clouds. Notice how they're drifting by without a care in the world. That's you right now - you don't have a care in the world either

36. Just watch the clouds constantly moving forward. Notice how the shapes keep changing. Also notice the images they create. Your life is like this - it keeps changing and moving forwards; even if you don't notice it

37. Now bring your attention back to your hammock. Slowly climb out of your hammock and walk back across the lawn to the water fountain. As you walk take time to notice all the beautiful colours in your garden

38. As you reach the water fountain look into the crystal clear water. Notice how soothing the running water is

39. Now focus on your breathing again

40. Breathe in deeply and then very slowly breathe out

41. Allow your breathing to bring you back to the room. Just keep breathing in deeply and breathing out slowly, but don't open your eyes yet

42. Gently bring your mind back to today and where you are. Feel yourself in the room, sitting in your chair

43. When you feel ready open your eyes. There's no rush

44. You're now back from your meditative journey

45. Sit quietly for a moment with your eyes open and allow yourself to readjust. How do you feel?

4.46 Shoulders, Arms And Neck Deskercises

Deskercise is a catchy name given to exercises that you can do at your desk. There are lots of different versions of deskercises available. These exercises are based on the deskercises created by author, Emily Milam. Each of these exercises is designed for the workplace, and takes just a few minutes.

We already know that physical exercise is beneficial in tackling stress. Research suggests that even deskercise can be beneficial to physical health and mental wellbeing. A short burst of deskercise will have some benefit if you're stressed as it will provide a welcome distraction for a few minutes.

Time required: 2-5 minutes per exercise

Instructions:

Your shoulders are the area that absorbs most tension. Therefore, some of these shoulders and arms exercises may be particularly helpful. You can do just one, some, or all three of these exercises; the choice is yours.

The Shoulder Shrug:
Simply raise both shoulders up toward your ears, hold for a count of 5 and then relax. Repeat this exercise for 2 minutes to release some of the tension in your neck and shoulders. If any worries pop into your head imagine yourself shrugging them off.

A Variation On The Push-up:
Stand one to two feet from the wall. Lean forward until your palms are flush against the wall, with your arms straight and parallel to the ground. Next, bend your elbows to bring your body towards the wall. Hold up to a count of 5 and then push yourself back to the starting position.

Repeat this exercise for 2 minutes. With each push, imagine yourself pushing your stresses and anxieties away. Repeat this exercise whenever you start to feel under pressure.

The Neck Strengthener:
Put your head in your hands as if exasperated by something or someone. Next, press your palms into your forehead as if trying to push your head backwards. Resist the motion by engaging you neck muscles. Hold up to a count of 5. Slowly relax.

Next, clasp your hands behind the back of your head and try to push your head backwards, resisting the motion with your hands. Hold up to a count of 5.

Repeat both parts of this exercise 5 times.

Any exercise that works on the neck is helpful as this part of the body often attracts stress.

4.47 Shoulder Stretch Exercise

This quick stress buster exercise can be done anywhere and at any time. All you need is an open doorway. This exercise will open up your chest, stretch your shoulders, and help remove some of the tension in your shoulders.

Time required: 2 minutes

Instructions:

1. Stand in front of an open doorway. With your right arm extended forward at shoulder height

2. Bend your elbow to make a right angle and lay your forearm upright against the door jamb

3. Lean into the open doorway while gently twisting your upper body away from your upraised arm. Hold the stretch for a count of 5. Relax and return to your standing position

4. Extend your left arm forward at shoulder height

5. Bend your elbow to make a right angle and lay your forearm upright against the door jamb

6. Lean into the open doorway while gently twisting your upper body away from your upraised arm. Hold the stretch for a count of 5. Relax and return to your standing position

7. Repeat this exercise for 2 minutes, or until you've had enough

4.48 Side Stretch Exercise

This quick side stretching exercise can be done anywhere (including your desk) and at any time. All you need is a chair and a couple of spare minutes. As part of this exercise you are going to release some of your worries.

Time required: 2 minutes

Instructions:

1. Sit tall in your chair, or stand up if you prefer

2. Stretch your arms above your head. Interlock your fingers and turn your palms to the ceiling

3. Breathe in deeply and exhale slowly

4. As you exhale, bend your body to the right side, still holding your arms above your head. Slowly return to the upright position

5. Take another deep breath. As you exhale this time bend your body to the left side, still holding your arms above your head. Slowly return to the upright position

6. Repeat this exercise for 2 minutes or until you've had enough. With each stretch release one of your anxieties. As you do so, say "work issues (or financial worries or whatever else is causing you stress) I release you"

7. When you return to you tasks try not to think about the issues you've just released

4.49 Stretching Exercise

Even a few minutes 'time out' can be calming and refreshing. You don't need to make big changes to the way you live your life. This stretching exercise doesn't cost anything to do and doesn't require any special equipment.

You can do this exercise as often as you like. Ideally, try to do this exercise once a day. It will help you to maintain a sense of wellbeing and keep your muscles relaxed. You can do this stretching exercise wherever you are. It takes just a couple of minutes but can help to give you a short energy boost.

Time required: up to 5 minutes

Instructions:

1. Put down anything you have in your hands. Stand up straight. You can do this exercise sitting down but it's more beneficial as a standing exercise

2. Place your feet a few inches apart and slightly bend your knees so you're standing firmly but not rigidly. As you stand, straighten your back and feel it gently stretching. Only stretch as far as feels comfortable. Hold to a count of 5. Now relax

3. Tip your head back slightly and look up at the ceiling (or sky if you're outside). Feel your neck stretching slightly. Hold to a count of 5. Now relax

4. Raise your right arm above your head as if you're reaching for something above you. If it helps imagine you're about changing a light-bulb, picking fruit from a tree or climbing a rope. Hold to a count of 5

5. Slowly bring your right arm down and let it drop by your side

6. Raise your left arm above your head as if you're reaching for something above you. Stretch as far as feels comfortable. Hold to a count of 5

7. As you stretch notice the movement undoing some of the tension in your neck

8. Slowly bring your left arm down and let it drop by your side

9. Alternating your arms, repeat this stretching exercise 5 times or until you feel more energised

10. Now tilt your neck to the right (as if you're trying to rest your head on your right shoulder). Hold this position to a count of 5

11. Slowly return your neck to its normal position

12. Tilt your neck to the left (as if you're trying to rest your head on your left shoulder). Hold this position to a count of 5

13. Slowly return your neck to its normal position

14. Repeat the neck tilting 5 times to the right and 5 times to the left

Note: Your neck may feel very stiff when you start this exercise. This is due to a build-up of tension in your neck and shoulders. The more you do this exercise the more flexible your muscles will become

15. Let both arms rest by your side, and straighten your neck

16. Give your arms and hands a quick shake. You are doing this to release some of the negative issues that you've been hanging onto. Now you're ready to resume your normal activities

Tip: If you feel silly doing this in front of other people at work, make it part of a team exercise.

4.50 Taking Control Of Stress Exercise

We all have preconceived ideas about our stressful situations. The purpose of this exercise is to help you get things into perspective. The aim is to help you break the cycle of self-fulfilling prophecy caused by negative thoughts. All you need for this exercise is pen and paper.

Stress is like a tiger; it's not the animal you're scared of it's what it could do to you!

Time required: 20-30 minutes

Instructions:

1. Write a list of all the things currently causing stress in your life. This will be a combination of major and minor stressors. Don't analyse them, just write them down

2. When your list is complete, choose just one stressor from your list

3. Write a detailed description of this stressor/stressful situation. Use single words or very short statements to describe the issue. Don't write lengthy sentences, but do make your description as detailed as possible

Note: The act of writing about this stressor is part of the clearing or getting things into perspective process

4. Create two columns on your piece of paper. The heading for column one is 'Can Control'. The heading for column two is 'Can't Control'

5. Look at your detailed description. Decide what you can control about this situation. Write a list of all the things you can control in column one

6. Now decide what you can't control about this situation. Write a list of all the things you can't control in column two

7. You should now have two lists. It doesn't matter if one is longer than the other

8. Look at the 'Can Control' column only for now. What actions you are going to take? Create an action plan. There's no point identifying what you can control if you don't do anything about it

9. Now look at the things you can't control. This is your reality check. You now have two choices. Your first choice is to accept that some things are beyond your control and not get stressed about it.

Alternatively you can give stress the upper hand and continue to fret and worry about the things you can't control. This is unhelpful, and may lead to physical health or emotional wellbeing issues. This may feel a little harsh, but this is the reality of your situation

10. Give yourself a pat on the back. You have taken some positive steps to reducing your stress level by gaining some control over this situation

Note: You can repeat this exercise for each of your stressors. Don't overload yourself by doing them all at once though. Overloading yourself simply adds to your stress level rather than reducing it.

If you feel tired after doing this exercise do something energising, like a stretching exercise.

4.51 Taoist Relaxation Technique Exercise

The Taoist Relaxation Technique is a good way to reduce pressure. If you do it regularly you will notice a difference. In fact, if you do this exercise daily you will start to notice changes within a week. The result will be a much less tense body.

Before you start this exercise decide whether you want to work with a golden light or a pure white light. Either is fine.

Time required: 15-30 minutes

Instructions:

1. Find somewhere quiet where you won't be disturbed. A bedroom is an ideal setting for this exercise. Switch off your mobile phone and switch the landline ringer off too

2. Lie on the floor/bed with your legs out straight and your feet slightly apart. Your arms should be straight by your sides and your palms facing upwards

3. Breathe in deeply through your nose. Hold your breath for a count of 3-5. Slowly exhale through your mouth

4. Repeat this breathing exercise for 2-5 minutes until you feel yourself starting to relax

5. You're now ready to start. As you inhale imagine a shaft of (gold or pure white) light flowing into your body through the crown of your head. With each inhalation you are going to focus on a different part of your body starting with your head

6. Breathe deeply and imagine your head filling with this beautiful light. With each in-breath see this light filling your head. Repeat this for 1 minute

7. With your next breath, imagine this light flowing moving down to your throat. With each in-breath see this light flowing to your throat. Repeat this for 1 minute

8. When you're ready, shift your attention to your chest. With each in-breath see the light flowing down through your head and throat into your chest. Repeat this for 1 minute

9. Breathe deeply again. Now imagine this light flowing into your body and moving down your arms and reaching your fingertips. With each in-breath see the light beginning its journey at your crown. See it travelling down through your body to your fingertips. Repeat this for 1 minute before moving on

10. Take another deep breath. Imagine this light flowing down to your solar plexus and stomach. Once again, see each in-breath starting at your crown. See this beautiful light flowing down to your stomach and solar plexus. Repeat this for 1 minute

11. When you're ready move on. Breathe in deeply and imagine this beautiful light moving down through your body. See it going down your legs and finally reaching your toes. As this light flows through the length of your body notice how completely relaxed you feel

12. You may choose to repeat steps 6-11, depending on how you feel

Don't rush this exercise as you want it to provide you with a deep sense of relaxation. By the time you reach your feet you should be feeling completely relaxed.

Note: You may find this exercise difficult at first. Your mind may wander back to your daily life or the things causing you stress. This is normal, and will happen less often as you become experienced at doing this. Simply acknowledge your thoughts, breathe in deeply and focus on that part of your body again.

4.52 The Calming Effects Of Colour Exercise

Research has shown that different colours have different effects upon us psychologically, emotionally and even physically. Therefore, it stands to reason that colour has a part to play in stress or stress management.

Some colours will have a negative impact on you and others will have a positive impact. Colour can be a great tool in your efforts to manage stress and feel more in control.

Colour therapy uses colour and light to balance energy wherever it's lacking in your body. There are many colour charts that you can find on the internet. You will find that they share similar evaluations about the effects of specific colours.

A very simple way to incorporate colour therapy into your life is through the clothes you wear each day. Simply listen to your intuition. Which colour do you feel you want to today?

Personally, I've been practising this type of colour therapy for many years. For example, I always wear a shade of blue if I have to give a presentation, or have a message to communicate.

Below is a summary of various colours and their effects on your physical and emotional wellbeing. You may think this is nonsense and has no merit. Try it before dismissing the idea.

Black: This can be an overpowering colour at times, as it exudes a feeling of power and elegance. It can also represent submission. In colour psychology black represents protection from external emotional stress.

Black creates a barrier between itself and the outside world. It provides comfort while protecting your emotions and feelings. Black is believed to be a good colour for hiding vulnerabilities, insecurities and lack of self-confidence.

Many people wear black to disguise their weight. Others use it to hide our feelings, fears or insecurities.

Blue: This is widely recognised as a tranquil colour. Blue has tremendous stress management qualities as it has the power to make you feel peaceful and calm.

From a colour psychology perspective, blue suggests reliable and responsible. Blue is a good colour to wear in difficult times. It represents order and direction, including living and work spaces.

Blue is also a good colour to wear when delivering presentations or public speaking as it promotes good communication.

Brown: This is a very important colour in terms of stress management. Brown is a very grounding colour. Brown is often viewed as being a comforting and stabilising colour. This may be just what you need to help deal with the stresses of modern life.

Gold: This is a feel good colour. It's a good colour to wear if you're feeling down and need to lift your spirits. Gold is viewed as the colour of success, achievement, triumph, abundance, prosperity, luxury, quality, prestige and sophistication.

Green: This is viewed as a restful, soothing and quiet colour that invites harmonious feelings. Green is a good colour for diffusing anxiety. Green relates to stability and endurance and is thought to provide persistence and the strength to cope with adversity. Wear green if you need help to concentrate on a particular task.

Grey: This is perceived as an unemotional, solid and stable colour. It's a useful colour to wear if you need to appear neutral or impartial. Grey can stifle and depress energy. If you're feeling hyper it can help to calm you down.

Indigo: This deep midnight blue is the colour of intuition and perception. It promotes deep concentration during times of introspection and meditation. Indigo helps you achieve deeper levels of consciousness. It also stimulates the right brain or creative activity.

As a colour, indigo conveys integrity and deep sincerity and so can be useful in stress management.

Magenta: This colour is useful if you need to raise your energy level. Magenta helps to create harmony and balance in every aspect of your life; physically, mentally, emotionally and spiritually. Magenta can be uplifting when you're unhappy, angry or frustrated.

Magenta can be a negative influence for some people. It can promote depression and despair in some, and prevent others from dealing with challenges. If it makes you feel negative avoid it.

Pink: This colour is most often associated with compassion, nurturing, love and emotion. Pink is seen as a soft and tranquil colour. Its peacefulness promotes a balance of your energies.

In colour psychology, pink is a sign of hope. It is a positive colour inspiring warm and comforting feelings, a sense that everything will be okay. Pink is a useful colour to wear if you feel in need of a little TLC.

Orange: Like red, orange is not a calming colour. Orange is a physically and mentally stimulating and intense colour. It can work to invigorate you when you are feeling low. On the converse side it's not a good colour to wear if you need emotional or physical soothing. Orange gets people thinking and talking so it's a good colour to wear if you're attending a networking event.

Red: This colour is not one to use for stress management. Red is an exciting and stimulating colour, usually associated with energy, passion and vigour. You might want to use red when you want to lift yourself out of an emotional slump or want to appear confident. Don't wear red if you're stressed and want soothing.

Silver: This is a soothing, calming and purifying colour. From a colour psychology viewpoint, silver signifies a time of reflection or change of direction.

Silver helps with cleansing and releasing mental, physical and emotional issues and blockages. It opens new doors and lights the way to the future.

Silver works well with most other colours as it illuminates and reflects the energy of those colours that surround it.

Turquoise: This colour will recharge your spirits during times of mental stress and tiredness. In colour psychology, turquoise controls and heals the emotions creating emotional balance and stability.

It is a great colour to help with clear thinking and decision-making. Turquoise assists in the development of organisational and management skills. It's a colour to wear if you want to influence others rather than preach or demand.

Violet: This represents strength, peace and wisdom. Violet can give you feelings of inner peace when you wear it as it's a relaxing and mind calming colour. Decorating with violet can give your personal space a peaceful feeling, relieving stress internally and externally.

White: White is symbolic of clarity and freshness. Wearing white will help to cleanse your mind. It really needs to be a clean, bright white. Once it gets dingy and dull your emotions can mirror the dullness.

Yellow: This is seen as a sunny and cheerful colour. It resonates with the left or logical side of your brain. Yellow stimulates your mental faculties and is helpful in creating mental agility and perception.

When you live in a positive state you are well-equipped to combat pressure and stress. Wear something yellow to lift your spirits.

If you have never worked with colour before I hope you will give it a try.

Time required: 10-30 minutes

Instructions:

1. Make a list of the colours that you most often wear. Why do you wear these colours? Next read the summary for each colour to identify your needs and how colour is helping you

2. Are there any colours that you are now going to incorporate into your life?

3. Make a note of any thoughts or feelings you have about particular colours. This will help to fine tune your awareness of the effect of colour on you

4. Think about ways to incorporate colour into your environment (home, workspace or garden etc)

5. You may like to revisit your notes in one, two and three months' time to see what has changed

4.53 The Letting Go Exercise

This exercise can be helpful if you're feeling very stressed as a result of a major trauma in your life. Unlike most of the exercises in this book this one could take weeks, months or years to complete. This is fine; simply add to it whenever you want to.

Time required: There is no defined timescale for this exercise

Instructions:

1. Get a large box or container, with a lid. It's important that your box has a lid

2. Give your box a name. You could name it 'My Higher Self', 'My Pain and Grief Box', 'The Source', or use the name of the person or situation that has caused the stress. There are no hard and fast rules here, simply give your box a name that works for you

3. Each time you're confronted with something that is bigger than you can handle write it down. Then put the piece of paper in the box

4. You may find inspirational cards that talk to you, or find items that invoke specific memories. These can go into your box too

5. If you're writing messages for your box, add as much detail as possible. This is part of the releasing process

6. When you put the paper into your box let go of all the thoughts or worries you had. Let your box own the worries now

7. By doing this you are handing responsibility to the Universe. You're trusting that you pain will be healed and things will be sorted out in the best possible way

Some people don't believe this exercise has any value. This is fine; after all one size doesn't fit all in stress management.

This exercise isn't a quick fix. Over time it will remove or reduce your stress and help you to adopt a more positive mind-set. This exercise works well for very serious stressful situations or trauma, like bereavement.

4.54 Visualisation Relaxation Exercise

We all have memories of feeling good. It can be a happy childhood, a particular event or experience, or just a period in your life when everything was going well. These thoughts invoke happy images in your mind. This is called visualisation.

Next time you're going through a stressful period in your life you may find it beneficial to do a visualisation exercise.

The aim of visualisation is to free your mind of the mental clutter. Don't worry if you struggle to keep you mind focused initially. This exercise gets easier and more effective the more you do it. It works best if you can do it in a fairly quiet place, without distractions.

You can do a visualisation exercise sitting down, standing or walking. It can be done anywhere, and at any time to suit you. For the purpose of this exercise I've chosen sitting on a chair.

Time required: 5-30 minutes

Instructions:

1. Sit down in a chair, with your back straight. Put your feet on the floor and rest your hands in your lap

2. Breathe in deeply through your nose. Hold your breath to a count of 3-5. Slowly exhale through your mouth

3. Let your breathing become slower and deeper with each breath. Repeat this deep breathing until you feel yourself starting to relax

4. Breathe in deeply and slowly exhale once more. As you breathe out this time feel your arms, legs and body become relaxed, and

know that you are perfectly safe and in control. You can open your eyes at any time

5. Continue to breathe in deeply and exhale slowly until your body feels completely relaxed

6. Each time you exhale let go of one problem in your life that is troubling you. If you can't let go of a particular thought make a mental note to deal with it later

7. Continue breathing in and out, and as you do so just let go of all your worries and anxieties

8. When you have managed to get rid of some of your emotional baggage you are ready to begin the visualisation. Visualise a happy memory. It can be something from your childhood, or an event or experience in your life (e.g. a wedding or party you've been to). It can be anything that brings happy thoughts into your mind

9. Visualise this image in as much detail as possible. Imagine you're describing it to someone and you want them to understand how magical this memory is. The more detailed your visualisation the better

10. Notice the sense of peace, tranquillity and contentment you're feeling right now. All your worries are gone for a little while. This is your relaxation time

If your mind wanders back to your day-to-day worries, just acknowledge them and return to your visualisation. With practice you will be able to block everything out apart from your visualisation

11. For a few minutes allow yourself to enjoy this experience. Feel it, smell it, hear it etc. Your day-to-day life seems so far away, and none of it matters right now. You can deal with it later

12. When you have finished your visualisation give it a name. Now focus on your breathing once more

13. Breathe in deeply and then very slowly breathe out

14. Slowly bring your mind back into the room. Just keep breathing in deeply and breathing out slowly, but don't open your eyes yet. Become aware of your surroundings. Feel yourself sitting in the chair

15. Allow your mind to come back to now

16. When you feel ready open your eyes. There's no rush, just open your eyes when you're ready to face the world again

17. Sit quietly for a moment with your eyes open and allow yourself to readjust. When you are ready resume your activities

18. You can bring the visualisation back to life anytime by simply remembering its name. As you remember the name you will begin to think about all your memories associated with it

4.55 Walking Meditation

Unlike other types of meditation, this one requires comfortable clothes and footwear, but doesn't involve sitting or lying down. As the name suggests, you're going for a walk.

Walking meditation is good for stress relief as it incorporates exercise and meditation. Simply build the meditation into your normal walk (with the dog, friends or on your own).

Time required: As long as you wish to walk. An hour is ideal as this gives the meditation time to really work for you

Instructions:

1. Before you start, give yourself permission to enjoy your walk. For this short time, don't worry about any of the issues in your life

2. Before you begin walking breathe in deeply through your nose. Hold your breath to a count of 3- 5. Exhale very slowly through your mouth

3. Repeat this breathing exercise for a couple of minutes until you feel yourself starting to relax. Now you're ready to begin your walking meditation

4. As you walk be aware of your body. Focus on lifting and placing each foot in front of the other. As you walk notice any sensations in your feet and legs. Are you feeling any sensations anywhere else e.g. you back?

5. As you walk, notice your surroundings, the birds, weather, scenery, traffic etc. Drive all other thoughts from your mind, and simply allow yourself to focus on enjoying your walk. If your mind strays simply refocus on your walking

6. Notice how you feel emotionally. Are you feeling light and carefree, or do you feel heavy?

7. At the end of your walk breathe in deeply through your nose. Hold your breath to a count of 3-5. Exhale very slowly through your mouth. Repeat this 3 times

8. Consciously say "goodbye walk" (out loud or silently) and then return to your normal activities

Note: If you were able to focus on your walk, energetically you will feel much lighter. Do a walking meditation as often as you are able to. With practice you will notice that during the walking meditation all you focus on is walking.

4.56 Walking And Writing Meditation

This is a walking meditation with an added element. Walking is widely recognised as being physically and emotionally beneficial, so build it into your life as often as possible.

You will need a pen and paper for this exercise.

Time required: As long as you wish to walk. An hour is ideal as this gives the meditation time to really work for you

Instructions:

1. Give yourself permission to enjoy this me-time

2. Before you begin walking, breathe in deeply through your nose. Hold your breath to a count of 3-5. Exhale very slowly through your mouth

3. Relax. Now you are ready to begin your walking and writing meditation. Before you set off, think of one of your stressful situations. Alternatively, do you have a problem/issue/question that requires some clear thinking?

4. Either out loud or silently, state the question or issue you need help with

5. Now begin your walk. As you walk focus on your legs and other parts of your body. Are you aware of any sensations? Don't think about your question right now - just walk

6. Enjoy your surroundings. Notice the sounds around you. Observe the scenery, the sky etc. Do you see any birds, wild animals or interesting landmarks?

7. Periodically stop. Think about your question/issue briefly and write down any observations you have. Don't analyse your thoughts; just write them down. Only spend a few minutes doing this

8. Resume your walk. Once again, focus on your surrounding and the act of walking. Don't worry about your question. Only think about your question/issue when you stop to make notes. By not focusing on the question/issue too much you allow your creative side to work its magic

9. Repeat steps 7 and 8 until you reach the end of your walk

10. At the end of your walk, breathe in deeply through your nose. Hold your breath to a count of 3-5. Slowly exhale through your mouth. Repeat this 3 times

11. Say goodbye to your walk

12. Review your notes/observations and decide what action you will take

13. Return to your normal activities

This is a good creative problem solving exercise as well as a useful stress management exercise.

4.57 Write A Letter Exercise

Some professionals say writing a letter you never intend to send is a good way to reduce stress and emotional intensity.

If you're feeling angry or upset write a letter to the person you're angry with. As you know you don't intend to send it, you can say everything you are feeling. Vent all your emotions; no matter how vitriolic. This exercise is about making you feel better afterwards.

Time required: No specified time

Instructions:

1. Write down everything you're feeling about the person or the situation

2. Put your letter somewhere safe for 24 hours. You don't want anyone to find this letter and read it

3. On day two read your letter and revise it to include any new thoughts you have

4. Put your letter somewhere safe for another 24 hours

5. On day three read your letter again. Have you included everything you want to say? Don't delete anything. These are thoughts you felt at the time of writing

6. When you're letter is complete burn it and watch the paper turning into ashes. Visualise the problem disappearing (going up in smoke metaphorically speaking)

7. Bury the ashes in the garden. If you don't have anywhere to bury the ashes it's OK to throw them in the bin instead

8. Give yourself permission to forgive and release the person or stressful situation

9. Allow your emotions to go. Remember, continuing to think about it simply increases the pressure you feel and doesn't make things better

4.58 Yogic Breathing Exercise

Yogic breathing is known to calm, soothe and de-stress you. Sometimes you don't have time for a full yoga session, or aren't interested in yoga. Here's a quick yogic breathing exercise developed by yoga expert, Emma Harding, at yogafix.com.

You can do this quick exercise while doing something else e.g. reading a magazine. "It's a simple and profound practice that helps still the mind, calm the nerves and give your brain a break" says Emma Harding.

Time required: 2 minutes

Instructions:

1. For this exercise we will imagine you're sitting down. Rest the back of your hands on top of your thighs

2. Breathe in deeply. As you do so, spread your fingers and palms as wide as possible

3. Slowly breathe out. As you do so curl your fingers in towards your palms

4. Repeat this exercise for at least 2 minutes or until you feel calm

"Sometimes when people are under stress, they hate to think, and it's the time when they most need to think" - Bill Clinton

5. Conclusion

According to Dr Aric Sigman it's good to have a bit of stress in your life. Personally, I'm not sure I agree that stress is good. I think what Dr Sigman refers to as good stress is what I call pressure i.e. challenges that inspire and motivate you. This helps to keep you healthy.

Being completely healthy means balancing your physical, mental and emotional wellbeing. It's not just a matter of a healthy diet and regular exercise.

The way you live your life, your behaviour, attitudes and personal habits, can have profound effects on your physical health. Your mind is constantly working at a rapid pace. This depletes its power, making it hard to focus and make the right choices in life.

To make up for what your body lacks your food is fortified with vitamins and minerals. Your mind also needs nourishing. If you fail to nourish and nurture your mind you open the door to stress.

During the course of my extensive research I kept coming across the same message "be kind to yourself". Stress is tough enough anyway, so don't add to it by being judgemental. Praise yourself for each step you take to reduce or remove your stress.

It's a fact, we are living in a 24/7 world. This is bound to create a level of stress as it means that downtime has to be consciously planned. What used to be described as a work/life balance is now referred to as a work/life merge. This can translate into stress if you don't carefully manage the two.

Are you one of those people who are always there to fix other people's problems? This could be your children, other family members, friends or colleagues. Stop! Before you can help anyone else you need to take care of you.

With over 170 exercise, strategies and techniques in this book I hope you found some suggestions to help you tackle your personal stress issues. Don't neglect yourself.

You may decide you don't have time for some of the exercises in this book. I have taken this into consideration and found a one-minute solution for you. Why not try one minute of silence?

Silence can be enormously beneficial to your emotional wellbeing. Try introducing one-minute breaks throughout the day to help you feel calm and in control? The following website has some free tools and suggestions to get you started - www.hydrateyourspirit.com.

I was prompted to research and write this book due to an overwhelmingly stressful period I was going through. The exercises that I've applied have definitely helped me to arrive at a much calmer place. I'm now better able to accept the things I can't control.

One thing I have definitely learnt is a positive mental attitude helps. The more positive your frame of mind the less stressed you will feel. Also, when stress does hit you will feel better equipped to cope with it.

If you haven't already created a personal action plan you might find it helpful to do so.

Finally, here are some additional websites that might interest you or help you in your quest to reduce your stress level.

The Global Retreat Centre - www.globalretreatcentre.com and www.bkwsu.org

The Stress Management Society - www.stress.org/uk

The International Stress Management Association - www.isma.org.uk

The Independent Mindfulness Information Website - www.minfulnet.org

Emily Milam (Deskercise creator) - www.greatist.com

You may have your own coping strategies and exercises. If you would like to share your ideas I would be delighted to hear from you. Please do get in touch - shepherdcreative0603@gmail.com.

Thank you for buying my book. I hope in some small way I've helped you deal with some of your stress.

"Stress is an ignorant state. It believes that everything is an emergency" - Natalie Goldberg (Wild Mind)

#0152 - 160117 - C0 - 210/148/8 - PB - DID1721749